MW00928181

Strong Hauler: Learning to live with Lo[ng]

Published by Ibral[...]

Visit the author's website at www.ibrahimrashid.com

Cover Design and Illustration by Margarita Louka
Edits by David Michael Chrisinger, Dr. Divya Jain, and Nicole Guenther

ISBN: 9798375690223

*Dedicated to my loving*

*mother, father, and sister,*

*who have always believed in me.*

# Table of Contents

Foreword 4

Introduction 6

RESILIENCE 10

Treat Long COVID like a Martial Art 11

Good Doctors will Empower You 13

Control Your Thoughts 17

Embrace Rest Early On 20

Work with Your Body 22

Food is Healing 25

You're Going to Lose Friends 27

Good Friends will Transform Your Health 30

Love Someone Good for your Nervous System 32

Work for Someone who will Treat You as a Partner 35

Show your Scars, but Don't Spill your Guts 37

Ask for Help and Tell People What You Need 39

Be Patient with Your Loved Ones 42

Lean on the COVID Long-hauler Community 44

Live in a Place Where You Can Happily be Ill 47

Find Meaning in Your Suffering 48

Give Yourself Permission to Cry 50

Take Your Mind to Space and Beyond 51

Let Go of Control 52

Write Down What You Love about Life 55

I'm Still Grieving 56

RELAPSE 58

Day 3: March 29, 2022      59

Supporting Another Survivor      63

Day 4: March 30, 2022      66

Letter from 2030 to the Present      69

Excerpt from a Friend's Diary      71

Day 5: March 31, 2022      73

Day 6: April 1, 2022      76

Day 7: April 2, 2022      80

Letter from 2035 to the Present      84

Supporting a Friend from Afar      87

Day 8: April 3, 2022      89

Day 9: April 4, 2022      91

Day 10: April 5, 2022      95

Day 11: April 6, 2022      98

Day 12: April 7, 2022      100

RECOVERY      102

Day 2: April 10, 2022      103

Day 5: April 13, 2022      104

Day 20: April 28, 2022      106

Day 28: May 6, 2022      107

Day 40: May 18, 2022      107

Day 48: May 26, 2022      108

Day 51: May 29, 2022      109

Day 64: June 11, 2022      109

Day 178: October 3, 2022      110

Acknowledgments      112

# Foreword

Dr. Peter Levine once wrote, "Trauma is not what happens to us, but what we hold inside in the absence of an empathetic witness." An estimated 12-25 percent of individuals faced with chronic illness experience a trauma response to their illness because their body no longer offers a sense of safety.[1] For these individuals, their worldview and sense of self, their existence as they have known it up till that point, have been shattered. For Ibrahim, his ability to achieve his academic and vocational potential seemed tenuous, and the mettle of the relationships that had filled his life with color were tested. There were times he wasn't sure that this journey of self-re-discovery was worthwhile. As many faced with chronic illness know, the daily struggle to survive and thrive despite our newfound physical, cognitive and/or mental health limitations can leave us feeling socially isolated when cherished others struggle to understand or empathize with our experience.

As his Clinical Psychologist, I have had the honor of bearing witness to Ibrahim's search for meaning as a COVID-19 long-hauler, and to be one amongst several who bolstered him when rehabilitative gains seemed to slip. In writing about his journey from surviving

---

[1] Edmondson, D. (2014). An enduring somatic threat model of posttraumatic stress disorder due to acute life-threatening medical events. Soc. Personal Pscyhol. Compass, 8(3), 118-134.

COVID-19 to thriving in spite of COVID-19, Ibrahim hopes to provide empathic support to others who are treading similar waters.

The process of writing this book has some interesting parallels to our therapeutic work together. Most apparent was finding the right balance between a mindset focused on hopes and possibilities and a mindset focused on the depth of one's struggles. Many of us have cultivated an outlook of toxic positivity to life that risks invalidating our internal experience. This approach is rewarded and reinforced by external messaging received from family and coworkers. Of course, there is another extreme of utter hopelessness that can be equally difficult to break away from. Discovering where we ought to land on the spectrum of hopefulness is an individual discovery process heavily influenced by one's socio-cultural context. Psychological therapy has been Ibrahim's outlet to discover the equilibrium that is right for him. This book is a reflection of his newfound balance, 100% authentic to his personal identity and values.

As a Clinical Psychologist, I know that any impact I have on a patient isn't always immediately apparent. It has been an eye-opening and likely a once-in-a lifetime opportunity to see the cumulative impact of our work come together in this unique manuscript. I hope that others feel heartened by Ibrahim's journey and find the needed support to continue their personal search for meaning so they too may learn to thrive despite chronic circumstances.

by Dr. Divya Jain, Psy.D
Chicago, IL
March 7, 2022

# Introduction

My name is Ibrahim Rashid and I am a COVID long-hauler. I moved to Chicago in October 2020 to start my master's degree at the University of Chicago. I was twenty-three, healthy without any preexisting conditions, and loved martial arts and skateboarding. By Halloween, I contracted COVID-19. The day Joe Biden won the American presidential election, I was in the emergency room. While people celebrated by Trump Tower, I waited for a physician to see me, unable to breathe.

The doctors said my case was "mild" and sent me home. They said I was fine. I wasn't. Over the next two years, I battled heart issues, brain fog, fatigue, chest pain, difficulty breathing, sleepless nights, joint pain, and reduced mobility. I lost friends, grappled with being disabled in the workplace, learned to use a cane, and struggled to continue graduate school.

I am one of the millions of people who never fully recovered from the virus. Battling this sickness has been the fight of my life. I almost gave up. But I didn't. I'm still here. Today, I am twenty-six years old, and I have learned to live with, rather than fight against, the effects of this virus. I can walk unassisted most of the time. I have a deeper relationship with my family; a robust support system of friends, faculty, mentors, coworkers, university staff, and well-wishers; and a loving partner. It's taken a while to get here, but for the first time in a long time, I have hope.

First of all, let me tell you what this book is not. This book is not a scientific exploration as to what Long COVID is or how to clinically treat it. People with more advanced degrees than I have are working on that. Rather, this book is a series of lessons I have learned along the way about how to keep on living when your world gets turned upside down.

In the first section of this book, titled "Resilience," each chapter is a lesson followed by an illustration of that lesson based on my own experiences. These are based on my reflections of the time between May 2021 and March 2022 after I lost my ability to walk and embarked on a radical journey of lifestyle changes to build resilience.

The "Relapse" section follows my twelve days in Spring 2022 when my symptoms came roaring back harder than ever before. In the third section "Recovery," I cover the aftermath of this challenging time. The first section is formatted as an advice column, while the second and third are my day-by-day thoughts as I navigate my first relapse.

I'll speak a lot about Long COVID and health within the context of my own experience because that is what I know. There will be times when I refer to the tests, treatments, medications, supplements, devices, and lifestyle changes I sought to manage my condition. I have an idea of what has helped me, but I cannot say for certain what will help you. The science on Long COVID is so nascent, after all. Of course, just because we currently do not know the causes of Long COVID and have yet to settle on a standard diagnostic test, does not mean we never will.

Some aspects of my recovery may not resonate with you. I have a robust health insurance plan. I was a graduate student at a selective and well-endowed institution, which afforded me access to resources and accommodations that others may lack. I was able to maintain my part-time, remote employment and receive financial support from my parents. I have certain forms of privilege that have benefited my recovery.

Moreover, each long-hauler has a different experience with the virus, which affects their response to different treatments. I was diagnosed with Long COVID five months after my initial infection but was never diagnosed with conditions like Chronic Fatigue Syndrome or Dysautonomia. My recovery plan focused largely on nutrition, rest, exercise, pacing, physical therapy, psychological therapy, and lifestyle change alongside some sedatives to dull my symptoms in the event of a relapse.

At the same time, I have met other long haulers who were infected before me, have taken many of the same steps as me, and have yet to improve. Few of us follow the same arc of recovery. So why write this book? For one reason: hope.

For two years, I believed that my condition would be permanent, and I would never get better. But then I did. I was able to go back to school and regain a semblance of normalcy in my life. I was able to fall in love and forge a stronger relationship with my family. I was able to bounce back from a terrible relapse and graduate. I was able to write this book and build my first company. I was able to *improve*. It still feels surreal to say that.

This book is for the long haulers out there looking for hope. By sharing my story with you, I seek to give you the emotional space needed to *believe* that things can get better.

# RESILIENCE

# Treat Long COVID like a Martial Art

I trained in Brazilian Jiu-Jitsu for two years before the COVID-19 pandemic. Jiu-Jitsu is a grappling-based martial art geared toward using an opponent's leverage and weight to bring them to the ground without landing a single kick or punch. I trained three to four times a week, visited academies whenever I traveled to new cities, and structured my entire social life around time on the mats.

Despite my efforts, I was not very good at it. I would get "submitted" (i.e., lose) while sparring against people with less experience than me. Everyone in my freshmen class got promoted and received stripes and colors on their belt, while I remained a novice white belt.

But I kept up with the sport. It showed me the limits of my body and how to overcome them. It surrounded me with a sense of community. My training partners and coach encouraged me to be the best version of myself both on and off the mats. Martial arts taught me that If I wanted to be a better fighter, I had to play a long game, analyze my successes and failures, and put in the work even when I felt like a failure. Most importantly, I simply loved the sport. It became a part of who I was.

When I found myself in a wheelchair in May 2021, my first thought was, "Will I ever fight again?" It seemed unlikely. That realization threw me into a pit of despair, where I felt as if I had lost a part of myself.

Then I paused and remembered my training. The martial arts teach you to breathe when you're stuck and create options for yourself. *I might not be able to physically do Jiu-Jitsu anymore*, I told myself, *but I'm still a fighter.* Jiu-Jitsu taught me to approach every day with gratitude, humility, perseverance, courage, and self-control.[2] I was determined to apply those lessons to my recovery.

I would structure my life around recovery and treat rest and healing like a full-time job that required preparation, the same way I structured my life around training. A year later, I realized that living with Long COVID and Jiu-Jitsu have a lot in common.

In both Jiu-Jitsu and Long COVID, there is pain, disappointment, and hopelessness. There are also small victories that come with discipline, iteration, and heart. When you first see someone fight, it looks like sheer madness. *How do they know when to strike or pounce? Will I ever be able to do that?* As you get more advanced, the logic starts to appear. Your body can do things that previously you could never imagine.

The same can be said for Long COVID. There is so much madness in dealing with this condition. No one really understands it yet. But with time and practice, you realize that, like martial arts, there is a playbook to managing your recovery. This book is my playbook.

_____

[2] This is the school creed of the Florian Martial Arts Academy in Boston, where I first learned Brazilian Jiu-Jitsu

## Good Clinicians will Empower You

Discovering you have Long COVID is quite a bizarre journey. You contract the virus, and once 14 days have passed, you start to feel fine. A few weeks or months later, you might notice that things are slightly off. Perhaps you wake up at night gasping for air. Maybe you can't read as much or work for as long as you used to. Or, like me, you have difficulty breathing, which will be bad enough that you'll pay a visit to a clinician. They give you some medication, run a few tests, and once the results come in, they tell you there is nothing to be worried about. *You are fine*, they say.

Confident in their assessment, you let a few months go by, ignoring the tightness in your chest and tickle in your throat, and you go about your life until again, you notice that things are off. But this time, things feel *really off*, and you find yourself struggling more than the first time around. Again, you go to a clinician and again, after running some tests, they might either say that there is nothing to be worried about, you are fine, and it's all in your head, or they may finally admit to you that they aren't sure how to explain your symptoms.

What happens next is crucial. You need to figure out if they are willing to be a partner in your health. You know your own body best. If things feel off and your clinician is dismissing your concerns, then run away from them as fast as possible. They're not helping you. Heck, they may just be giving you the runaround by making you do all sorts of tests that insurance may or may not cover. If you find yourself in this situation, please ask other long haulers for insight on who can help you. The Long COVID clinics can take months to get into, and they may not specialize in your specific ailment, so it is important to ask other long haulers for advice. You can connect with them through support groups like Body Politic or other advocacy groups.[3]

If you find a clinician who is willing to work with you through the uncertainty, stick with them. If you're part of the first few waves of COVID long haulers, as I am, then you're a guinea pig. No one knows how to treat us, so it is key to find someone who will not dismiss your concerns, are willing to explore and learn with you, and exemplify compassionate care. I have found two such clinician. The first was Terry Moore, a Neuromuscular and Cardiovascular Physiologist based in Canada who specialized in treating concussions and other complex illnesses. Through my friend, Spencer, I learned that Terry had experience treating symptoms like brain fog, fatigue, and immobility, even if they weren't directly caused by COVID.

During our first remote session together in July 2021, he spent three hours validating my experience. His theory was that coronaviruses caused muscles to contract. When they did so, they could push up against the nerves. This resulted in either a "pinch" which causes pain, or a "block" that cut off the nerve signal,

---

[3] The COVID-19 long-hauler Advocacy Project has created a COVID Competent Healthcare Provider list that you can access from here:
https://docs.google.com/spreadsheets/d/1qRz6jcMX2Yx7_prnJqdBQFXgVJE_CgZSlIYNs hW3XJM/edit#gid=718047883

rendering patients like me immobile, fatigued, or in pain. These pinches and blocks can be exacerbated by stress or poor sleep hygiene, which causes the muscles to suddenly contract or remain in a tighter state.[4] Terry has prescribed me a range of exercises and lifestyle changes to manage my symptoms, and he's helped me understand the mechanics of what is going on inside my body.

The other provider was my clinical psychologist, Dr. Divya Jain. Initially, I was searching for any health psychologist with clinical experience treating Long COVID. I was drawn to Dr. Jain because of our shared background as South Asian Americans. Dr. Jain helped me better understand the potential role of emotional and relational stressors in triggering some of my symptoms. She also helped me improve my meditation practice, develop stronger breathing habits, learn progressive muscle relaxation techniques that can help ease the tension in my body, and held me accountable as I've tried to incorporate Terry's recommendations into my new lifestyle. She taught me to silence my inner critic, calm my thoughts, and come to peace with my circumstances.

For both Terry and Dr. Jain, I was their first Long COVID patient. Neither of them gave up on me. Having a team of clinicians who will not only empower you with knowledge on how to take

---

[4] I must acknowledge that there is a wide variation of symptom experiences for each long-hauler, which means that different treatments might have varying levels of effectiveness. My experience is unique to me, and this is my interpretation of the explanation I was provided that has informed my own recovery.

ownership of your health, but who are also brave and humble enough to learn alongside you, is key to managing your illness.

# Control Your Thoughts

When you spend a lot of time sick and staring at the ceiling, it's easy to spiral into a series of destructive thoughts. Those thoughts, I realized early on, were having a detrimental effect on my wellbeing.

I came across *The Mind-Body Cure: Heal Your Pain, Anxiety, and Fatigue by Controlling Chronic Stress* by Dr. Bal Pawa, MD.[5] Dr. Pawa calls upon readers to see the "Mind" and the "Body" as one interconnected unit known as the Mind-Body. Mental health could affect your physical health, and vice versa. Taking ownership of your thoughts could ease your pain and promote healing, she reasoned. Each chapter of Dr. Pawa's book explores how stress, and its subsequent cortisol response, can affect a different part of the body. For example, chronic stress could cause bone decay, difficulty breathing, and muscle tightness and immobility.

If I couldn't take control of my body, I was determined to take control of my mind. I soon read the *Untethered Soul* and came across a profound idea. *You are not your thoughts; you are simply the observer of your thoughts.*[6]

---

[5] You can purchase the book here:
https://www.amazon.com/gp/product/B08J8LHJ54/
[6] It's a bit of a complicated idea. VaccusMonastica explains it in an intuitive way on Reddit: "You are the sky. Thoughts and feelings are the clouds. Clouds form [then dissipate]. You, the sky, remain. Thoughts and feelings are things you have. They are not what you are unless you decide to attach [a certain feeling, thought, or meaning to it].
https://www.reddit.com/r/Mindfulness/comments/5viu1a/you_are_not_your_th oughts/

This meant that I had to learn to have an *awareness* of my thoughts and the trains they could potentially take me on and build the power to pause and choose whether that's where I wanted to go.

If a thought came into my head that told me I was worthless, unlovable, deserving of my sickness, and doomed to be bedridden, I had to stop, breathe, and *choose* whether I wanted to entertain that thought or let it dissipate. In the early days, I spent a lot of time bedridden, depressed, and angry. I had to choose to let go of all the anger and ideas I had for myself that were weighing me down and making me sick.[7]

This meant I had to change my perception of time and let go of the timeline I had created for myself. A fellow long-hauler once told me that, "You do not control when you are done with the condition; the condition decides when it is done with you." It was a hard pill to swallow, but it's what I needed to hear.

I returned from the emergency room in May and dropped down to only one graduate course during the Spring Quarter of my first year, delaying my graduation by a whole quarter. I had to accept that my degree would take longer than most, and that was okay.

I also had to let go of my perception of what I thought my body should be. I held on so tightly to this image of myself as healthy

---

[7] Dr. Jain recommended this video to me, "Stop Overthinking: Leaves on a Stream ACT Anxiety Skill #30," to help practice calming my thoughts and quieting my mind. I listened to it every morning during the summer that I dedicated myself fully to rest. https://www.youtube.com/watch?v=vjKltKKSur8

and with the same physical abilities as my pre-COVID self. I was, after all, a skateboarder and a martial artist.

Holding on to this fixed image of who I thought I was only made me angry when my recovery wasn't as fast as I wanted it to be. *If I wasn't perfectly healthy, then I was a failure,* I told myself.

I worked to let go of these thoughts and adopt a "growth mindset" as opposed to a "fixed" one as it related to my health. A growth mindset is one in which you compare your health *today* to what it was the day before and celebrate your *progress* as well as your potential. A fixed mindset is one in which you focus on simply not being sick. By taking ownership of my thoughts, and letting go, I could begin the journey of restoring my health.

That is, of course, easier said than done. You cannot merely "forget" your problems in an instant. Anyone that says so embodies "toxic positivity." Prior to COVID, I attended therapy at different stages of my life and resumed my sessions during my recovery. Despite that prior inner work, I still struggled with these principles. This has meant that a large focus of my recent therapy journey with Dr. Jain has focused on having better inner dialogue, developing awareness of my thoughts and how it makes me feel, and finding acceptance with my condition. I do not believe that we can just switch on and off our negative feelings like a light switch. Rather, we can learn to improve our inner dialogue and be gentler with ourselves when faced with negative thoughts.

# Embrace Rest Early On

Early on in my health journey, I came across a blog post written by someone with Chronic Fatigue Syndrome (CFS), shared in the Body Politic Long COVID support group. It was titled "Indefinitely ill - Post COVID Fatigue."[8] Her message to COVID long haulers was to embrace rest early on, rather than powering through the illness. Her warning, based on her own experience with another post-viral illness, was that failure to slow down and focus on recovery *early on* would exacerbate the condition, and potentially make it permanent. Her message scared the living crap out of me.

I discovered that I didn't actually know how to rest or slow down. Was I supposed to just lay down in bed, sit in the dark, and stare at the ceiling all day? Doing so just made me feel even more depressed. It wasn't restorative at all. I moved in with my aunt and cousin in Michigan and began exploring what it truly meant to slow down and rest. I realized that rest was a function of energy. To be well rested, we need to minimize exposure to the things that drain us and immerse ourselves in whatever is replenishing.

During that summer, I told many of my friends that I would be unresponsive for a while; I needed the quiet just to think. In this period of trying to center my needs, I ended relationships with some people who were dismissive, mean, and draining. I spent a lot of time

---

[8] See here: https://crookedtimber.org/2020/05/18/indefinitely-ill-post-covid-fatigue/

lying in bed or sitting in the grass, listening to white noise or meditative music. I played catch with my cousin, took him to the pool, and introduced him to Star Wars. I spent time in the sun. I colored. And I took naps. Lots and lots of naps.

I began tracking my sleep. I purchased a WHOOP, a wearable device that many athletes use to figure out how much rest and activity they should undertake. The device works by assigning a "Recovery Score" that tells the user how well-rested their body is, based on factors such as heart rate and sleep quality.

I used the recovery score to figure out how much rest I needed to build into my day. If the WHOOP's Sleep Coach told me to sleep at a certain time to get "peak sleep performance," that's when I slept. If it told me that I had accumulated a sleep debt, I would build in exactly that amount of time for a nap.

It also showed me, through its habit tracker and analytical reports, how my lifestyle decisions were affecting my recovery and sleep scores. Taking melatonin, sleeping with a weighted blanket, taking baths in Epsom salts, using a humidifier, taking magnesium supplements, hydrating frequently, having consistent bed and wake up times, and stretching before sleeping all had a positive effect on my sleep quality and recovery score. Long COVID taught me how to rest for the first time.

## Work with Your Body

One morning, I woke up with a low recovery score on my WHOOP, which suggested that I should take it easy, but I was determined not to let the number determine what I did that day. I went for a swim in the evening, and as I was walking home, my knees started throbbing. I started dragging my feet and losing my balance. It was pouring rain, and I found myself lying on the ground, covered in mud, forcing myself to stretch so I could regain my balance. I was in tears. *I hate my legs so much. I hate how I can't walk. I hate this pain. I want it to stop.* I imagined how much better life would be if I didn't have my legs. *Surely, it would be better than this.* I stopped and caught that thought. I knew I didn't mean it. I took a series of deep breaths, sang Eminem's "Lose Yourself" to myself, stretched, got back up, and made it home.

Later that week, I talked about this episode with Dr. Jain in our therapy session. *My legs don't move as well as they used to*, I told her. Sometimes, I would try to push my body beyond its limit out of anger. I would try to bike faster than what I knew I could handle as a way to prove to my legs that I was better than them. I was disassociating my consciousness from my body.

But that was wrong, Dr. Jain reminded me. Our legs are what allow most of us to experience the world. They take us from place to place, allowing us to see our friends, meet our families, see new sights, and explore new cultures. Our legs are a part of our bodies, and our bodies carry our spirits that make us who we are. Thus, we need to treat our bodies with love, compassion, and care. It's taken me a while to realize that my body has fundamentally changed since I contracted COVID. Even though my body feels different, I need to love my body and find a way to work in partnership with it.

That has meant listening to my body when it sends me signals that my mind has yet to process. If I feel tired, I must rest. If my eyes are hurting, I should look away from screens. If my legs are aching, I should sit down and stretch. If my chest hurts, I should take some deep breaths.

If my body doesn't do what I want it to do, that's okay. I should be gentle with it and find a way to work with it. For example, I used to feel a lot of shame when I started using a cane. I hated appearing so visibly disabled. I could feel people's pity when they looked at me and remembered that I was the one who would rally all my classmates to go ice skating during the Chicago winter. It was worse when passengers refused to make space for me to sit in public transport, doors would be slammed in my face, I would be shoved in hallways, or when people at restaurants would directly ask me, "Why do *you* need this cane?" They probably assumed that because I looked young, I was faking it. This fueled all sorts of self-loathing and shame, directed toward my legs, when really, the problem was our society's internalized ableism and collective cruelty.

I had to learn to let my self-loathing go. As Terry taught me, getting angry and upset was only going to worsen my symptoms. I had to accept my new limitations, show love to my body, and start to see my cane as merely a tool that could help me experience life.

In coming to peace and acceptance with my body, I could start learning to work within my limits, and not push myself beyond what I knew I could handle.

# Food is Healing

In my first apartment, my roommates and I stuck the side of a McDonalds bag onto our wall and would add a tally underneath the golden arches whenever one of us would order fast food. Every time we ordered fast food, we had to draw a new tally line. Whenever I felt sick, I would order fast food. If I was in the emergency room, I'd order a Big Mac to be on my doorstep by the time I got home. If I was sick in bed for a week, I would subsist on chicken nuggets and fries.

My roommates could tell if I wasn't okay simply based on the new tallies on the wall. And I wasn't. The more I ate, the worse I felt, triggering a dangerous spiral. I realized that I had a problematic relationship with food, which was making me feel bad about myself, when I was already feeling sick. I needed to change. I learned that while our DNA provides the blueprint for *how* our body should be reproduced, the food we consume provides the "parts" that go into recreating us. Thus, what we put into our mouths can affect how our bodies are recreated, giving food restorative properties that can change how we feel.

It was time to transform my relationship with food from viewing it as a means of sustenance to treating it as a source of nourishment and healing. This is admittedly an area that I continue to struggle with. Generally, I'm trying to cut down my added sugar and processed food consumption because I've noticed that my legs always hurt afterwards. In addition, I'm trying to try new vegetables, eat fruits instead of candy, drink water when I face sugar cravings, and explore "Mediterranean Diet" recipes. It's not a lot, but my perception is that it has helped avoid me some unnecessary symptom spikes.

# You're Going to Lose Friends

I started writing this book in December of 2021, a little over a year after I contracted the virus. If you told me that some of the people who I called my "best friends" back in 2020 would no longer be around, I wouldn't have believed you. But unfortunately, the saying is true: you learn who your friends are when you are most in need. This year I lost several friends whom I thought I would hold onto for life, whom I envisioned would be at my wedding and would someday meet my future children.

One of these former friends I will call Alex. Alex and I had known each other for a few years, having gone through similar life milestones together. We had been each other's anchor as we both navigated post-college adulthood. She lived in a warmer environment than Chicago, and in spring 2021 I asked if I could stay with her for a week while I rested from a bout of intense sickness.

I explained that my bandwidth and health were low, and I just needed a supportive friend and warm environment. She obliged. On my second day in her home, I started feeling sick, possibly an effect from having just received my first dose of the COVID vaccine. That night, she told me I was a "buzzkill" who was ruining the "happy and therapeutic environment" in her apartment. She asked me to leave. As I left the next morning, I told her that I needed a pause from our friendship while I worked through my recovery and that I would reach out once I felt better. Months later, when I was in better health, I tried to reestablish contact. She didn't respond.

This has, unfortunately, played out with a lot of different people, and I sometimes struggle to reconcile why it happens. I've fallen into a spiral of destructive thoughts many times over this, wondering: *Is my illness that much of a burden? Should I bottle this all up, and keep it to myself? Why does no one care enough to understand what I'm going through? Why is no one ever there for me, in my intense moment of need, when I've always shown up for them?*

Dr. Jain and my first therapist, Dr. Wilczynski, helped me silence these questions, calm my head, and put things into perspective. The truth is that some people are just not equipped to handle illness, trauma, or tragedy. It overwhelms them. It also completely conflicts with the image they have of the newly ill person.[9] I once was an energetic, carefree person. COVID has completely changed who I am. It has realigned my priorities. I'm a lot more risk-averse, reserved, and to be honest, morbid.

There are times when I am honestly one of the most boring people around. I don't want to go out. I don't want to try new restaurants or go on hikes. All I want to do is rest, sit in the sun, and talk. I'm a different person now, who no longer fits the place they once put me in their life. So, they cast me aside. I've found peace with that.

COVID has also taught me to be a lot more intentional about with whom I spend my time with to be attuned to how they make me

---

[9] I do believes that because our society teaches us to devaluate disabled people's lives, it makes people unwilling to make accommodations.

feel. While there are some people who are simply incapable of seeing you at your lowest, warts and all, there are others who are willing to help pull you out of your lowest lows. It's important to focus on the people who are there, rather than those who have left you behind. You must come to terms with the fact that you will lose friends, and that's okay. It really sucks though.

# Good Friends will Transform Your Health

2021 was a year I lost some of my closest friends, but it was also the year I gained several deeper ones. Spencer Gudewill is one of the new people who have changed my life.

Two years ago, during his first month of graduate school, Spencer suffered a concussion while playing flag football. Like me, he went through waves of illnesses, lost friends, changed relationships, hopelessness and despair, and missed family outings and life events, all while trying to juggle his graduate studies.

He was the one who told me about the disability accommodations process at the University of Chicago and was the reason why I have more time on my tests, flexibility with my deadlines, and priority registration to build a schedule that works best to accommodate my fatigue and brain fog. He was the one who introduced me to Terry. He gave me books that helped me think of my disability as a strength, rather than a weakness.[10] And he has been a constant source of companionship for me during each step of my health journey. In fact, we have taken some of the same classes

––––––––––––––––––––––––––––

[10] Some might argue that there is a strand of "body positivity" that is counterproductive and dehumanizing, and that rather than viewing our ailments as a strength, we should view them neutrally. I recognize but disagree with this view. I think of what I have gone through as a strength. It has given me the courage to share my story, have a better view of myself, and cope with the lowest moments of this illness.

together and supported one another whenever the other fell behind because of their illnesses.

I do not know if I would be as healthy as I am today had it not been for him. Spencer is someone whose friendship has single handedly carried me in my recovery further along than anyone else. Illness will teach you that the friends you keep can literally transform your health. The same can be said for love.

# Love Someone Good for your Nervous System

Let's be honest, falling for someone is terrifying, no matter how old you are or what you've gone through. I realized early on that my Long COVID symptoms were triggered by emotional exertion. Being vulnerable and communicating boundaries and expectations with friends would cause me chest pain. Anger would trigger my brain fog. Being ghosted by a girl (after what I thought was a great date!) would put me in bed for days. Many long haulers suffer from Chronic Fatigue Syndrome (CFS) and describe these episodes as "crashes" or *Post-Exertion Malaise*.[11] I described them as the reason I couldn't date; I was too scared of what opening myself up to love would do to my fragile body – until I met Yasmeen.[12]

Yasmeen and I met the same way most young adults meet these days. We met online. We were both first year graduate students at the University of Chicago, and connected in a group chat when I asked if anyone knew where I could find a tattoo artist who had

---

[11] I never received a formal diagnosis of Chronic Fatigue Syndrome. I was told that you need to be experiencing symptoms for at least 6 months. I saw a neurologist at the five-month mark for my legs. At the time, I suspected that I did have CFS, but couldn't get a diagnosis because of how long I had been experiencing symptoms for. I never sought a second opinion once I did cross the six-month mark. At that point, I was too demoralized to see another doctor and didn't think a diagnosis would give me anything useful.

[12] Yasmeen is a pseudonym for my partner. Unfortunately, dating is considered taboo in American Muslim culture. I use a pseudonym to protect our relationship from familial and communal pressure.

experience with the Urdu-Arabic script.[13] She's Arab American and wanted to know the same thing. We traded some messages and called a few times over the next few months, but never consistently. She was studying remotely from out-of-state, and I was sick in bed barely able to handle school in Chicago.

In May 2021, when I suddenly found myself unable to walk and in the emergency room, she reached out, and we video called for the first time. Over the next few months, as I dropped several classes and moved to stay with my aunt in Michigan to focus on my recovery, she would check in constantly. A few texts turned into a few calls, which turned into whole nights over FaceTime. She was patient with me as I slowly opened up, sharing how hard it was to deal with this illness. Many people would tell me just to *be strong*. She would tell me that it's okay that I'm struggling and that she believed in me. She gave me the space to be vulnerable in my lowest moments.

When we shared our feelings for one another (or, as she likes to call it, opened our "can of worms"), I told her that I needed a partner who would not give up on me when I fell ill. I had already been abandoned by people before. I wasn't prepared to go through that again. She understood, and over the next few months, once we both returned to Chicago, she became my biggest advocate, best friend, and source of support.

---

[13] Urdu, which is one of the official languages of Pakistan and my mother tongue, has the same script as Arabic, save for a few letters.

By then, I had started using a cane and was trying to regain my mobility. She would leave social events with me when I told her I was getting ready to leave because people kept asking about my cane, I couldn't find a place to sit, or my legs were hurting. I would sometimes have to lay down on the ground to stretch or breathe because I suddenly lost balance, and she would sit next to me, whispering in my ear, *You're strong; you got this.* She would help me meal prep for the week when I was too weak to cook for myself. When I fell ill right before the flight to my cousin's wedding, she moved heaven and earth to help me pack, get ready, and make my way to the airport. I'm very grateful for her.

## Work for Someone who will Treat You as a Partner

Most people spend at least a third of their weekdays in the workplace. Our coworkers and the people we work for can have a profound effect on our wellbeing. As a long-hauler, I have found it incredibly valuable to foster open dialogue early on with my employers about what I'm going through, so I can create a supportive environment where I can both advance my recovery and achieve my professional goals.

In February of 2021, I was offered a summer internship to join a prestigious investment firm working in sustainability and finance. I saw this position as an on-ramp to the career that I wanted. When I lost my ability to walk a month before the start of my internship, I visualized waves washing away the sandcastle I was trying to build. Through LinkedIn, I met an openly disabled woman on the firm's team. I told her that I didn't know how to talk about my condition with my prospective supervisor. I was terrified that I would have to forfeit my position.

When we spoke, she encouraged me to view myself as "newly disabled," taught me about the Americans with Disabilities Act and the protections it afforded me, and she helped me think about how to disclose my disability and seek accommodations from HR and my supervisor. Later, she became my unofficial peer-mentor who helped me navigate my internship with a new illness.

I let HR and my supervisor know what had happened soon after our conversation. During my first meeting with my supervisor, she told me that she viewed my internship as a "partnership" that should be "mutually beneficial." My health, she affirmed, should always come first. If I ever needed to take a break, work a flexible schedule, or change my scope of work, she would accommodate me.

It's so important to work for someone who is willing to meet you where you are. I experienced that same level of respect and trust when I returned to IFF, a Community Development Financial Institute that provides debt financing to nonprofits in the Midwest, in the fall of 2021. I was working under Yi when I first started having difficulty walking and had to drop several of my classes. She saw my health transform overnight in the spring.

By fall, my number one priority was to figure out how to return to full time status at school, so I could continue to make progress on my degree while still balancing my recovery. I approached Yi with my desire, and she was willing to work with me to create an "independent study" that treated my work with IFF as my third course, enabling me to enroll as a full-time student. Yi was also someone who was willing to give honest and constructive feedback when I fell short – which I did often. I really struggled that quarter to balance school, work, and my health, and Yi would gently call me out on it and coach me on how to manage everyone's expectations, including my own.

I spent a lot of time early on in my recovery wondering whether and how I'll ever work again. But my coworkers and supervisors, especially Yi, all taught me how to return to the workforce and balance my recovery by treating me as a partner, and for that I'll always be grateful.

## Show your Scars, but Don't Spill your Guts

As I embarked on my job search for other internships and post-grad employment, I wasn't sure whether, or even how, to talk about what I had gone through. On one hand, I was scared to share my experience for fear of discrimination. On the other hand, I knew just how transformative having a supportive supervisor was for my well-being, and I told myself that if a company wasn't willing to meet me where I was at, they weren't worth my labor.

As terrifying as it was, I would make it a point to talk about my experience during interviews with potential employers. After all, interviews are a two-way street, where candidates are also assessing whether a company is a good fit for them.

When interviewers would ask me what my strengths are, I would tell them that I am resilient. I would then explain all the different ways I have worked with my body to improve my health. When people would ask me what my weaknesses are, I would explain that I'm learning to manage a complex illness that can sometimes cause me to become immobile or bed ridden. I would explain the different ways I try to mitigate these crashes (through symptom tracking, focus on sleep hygiene, meditation, supplements, etc.) but that sometimes I would need a buffer and flexibility. Upon disclosing, some people would awkwardly change topics, while most would empathetically listen and show curiosity.

When people ask me how I juggle multiple competing priorities, I talk about the concept of "pacing" and managing my "energy envelope," which is a technique that many in the Long COVID community use. I talk about how my health can deteriorate if I'm not well-rested or am overburdened, which forces me to plan my schedule weeks in advance; stick to a routine; inject joy, rest, and sunlight into my day; and take care of my mental, spiritual, and physical health.

I have since learned to recognize my condition for what it is— a source of strength, and proof of my resilience, rather than a liability. When I talk about it, I'm metaphorically looking someone in the eye, rolling up my sleeve, and showing my scars. I share the wisdom I've gained from my battle with Long COVID, as opposed to spilling my guts.[14]

---

[14] I was interviewed for an article in the MIT Sloan Review about "How Managers Can Support Employees with Long COVID" by Fiona Lowenstein where I expand upon some of the ideas mentioned in this chapter.
https://sloanreview.mit.edu/article/how-managers-can-support-employees-with-long-covid/

## Ask for Help and Tell People What You Need

As isolated as I often felt, I learned that I did not need to battle Long COVID alone. There were countless people around me who wanted to help. It's important to tell them what I need and lean on my community.

When I first lost my ability to walk, the doctors in the emergency room did not know what to do. They told me to take pain killers, go home, and try to find a neurologist. I was so demoralized. My parents asked my uncle in Pakistan, who is a physician, for help identifying a neurologist in Chicago. Later that night, I posted in the Slack channel of the American Pakistan Foundation:

> @Channel As of Wednesday, I've suddenly lost the ability to walk, and spent the last few days in the ER. Everything looks structurally fine, but I'm now in a wheelchair, and can stand with much difficulty.
>
> It's somehow COVID related... Currently struggling to find a Neurologist who can see me. Appointments are booked 2 months out. Does anyone have any leads? thanks all for your help and keep me in your duas [prayers] this Ramadan.[15]

---

[15] Ramadan is the holiest month of the Islamic Calendar in which Muslims believe the Quran, our holy book, was revealed by God. We observe Ramadan by daily acts of charity, immersing ourselves in prayer, and abstaining from food, drink, and sex

Over the next 48 hours, I kept getting calls from physicians around the country, offering advice, and trying to identify people within their network who could help me. Eventually, one of my uncles' nieces (who was a member of the American Pakistan Foundation) told her father, who was once a professor at a medical school in Pakistan. He told his former student, who connected me with a neurologist in Chicago. I left the emergency room on Thursday and saw that neurologist on Monday. I'll always be grateful for my family's help, and the American Pakistan Foundation's support, in helping me find a physician in my moment of need.

Throughout my health journey, I learned time and time again that if I just asked for help, I usually would receive it. Classmates would help me catch up on missed lectures. Friends would offer to bring me groceries. Their parents would make me food. Employers would make accommodations, and professors would provide extensions.

There were also some people who did not care what I was going through. They looked down upon me, dismissed my concerns despite me pleading for their assistance, and put up barriers that made situations worse. Still, I have found that if I ask people for help and tell people what I need, I receive that and more.

---

from sunrise to sunset for thirty days. We believe that in this month, God is listening most closely to our prayers.

40

I encourage you to think about moments where you have needs that you do not voice and reflect on how you might build the ability to ask for what you need. This requires vulnerability and overcoming the fears that they might say no or judge you for asking. In my experience, it is worth the risk.

# Be Patient with Your Loved Ones

It is easy to believe that you are the only one suffering through your sickness. After all, you are the one who had to slow down your degree. You are the one who spent months in therapy. You are the one who feels pain on a daily basis. You are the one who feels hopeless, wondering whether you will ever overcome this.

Most of these feelings are valid, except for one. You are not the only one suffering. Your family, and those who truly love you, are suffering alongside you, but in a different way. That took me a while to realize. There were times when I would talk to my parents and sister about what I was going through, and how hopeless and upset I felt, and they would shut down the conversation. They would tell me that they didn't want to hear about it because it made them sad. I used to get upset because I wanted to open up to my family. Their rejection made me feel like they did not care to hear what I was going through.

One day, while arguing with my dad about exactly this point, he said to me, "Do you realize how depressing it is that out of everyone who got COVID in our extended family, you, my son, are the one who has struggled to recover for more than a year? Have you ever thought about what it's like to watch this as a parent?" I'll be honest, I never did.

In focusing on my own pain, I somehow forgot that my parents flew halfway across the world when I lost my ability to walk, accompanying me to the doctor, helping me find physicians, paying for therapy, staying with me while I lived with my aunt, and being present every step of the way. That must have been so incredibly difficult and involved sacrifices I did not have the capacity to notice.

*I've realized that my parents do know what I'm going through.* They have seen it firsthand. They have seen who I was before, and who I am now, trying to rebuild my life. Their hearts break the most when they see just how much I struggle. Their hearts get filled with the most pride as I overcome each setback. They also feel the most helpless when doctors and they themselves do not know how to treat this condition, or when it will subside.

That's a difficult situation to be in, and that makes them act in ways that I may occasionally disagree with. In realizing that, I have had to learn to be patient with them and acknowledge that they are struggling alongside me.

# Lean on the COVID Long-hauler Community

Very few people will know exactly what you're going through. Those closest to you will develop some sort of an idea of what Long COVID feels like. Anyone who has ever experienced a complex or chronic illness will relate to you a bit more. But the people who can really understand what you're going through and empower you are your fellow long haulers. Finding them, especially those who you can trust, will be a lifeline.

I am lucky to have found other long haulers who were further along their journey, early on in my own illness. In the Spring of 2020, the University of Chicago experienced a rapid surge of the Delta variant due to an off-campus fraternity party, which shut down in-person classes for two weeks. During that time, I published an Op-ed in the school paper sharing my experience as a COVID long-hauler and called upon the University to make plans to educate students in isolation housing about Long COVID. I also wrote about how the University could better care for students if their symptoms persisted, as mine did. My article went viral and got me an audience with the University's senior leadership, who implemented many of my proposed reforms.[16]

---

[16] Rashid, Ibrahim, "After COVID: Advice from a Long-Hauler," The Chicago Maroon, April 9, 2021.  https://www.chicagomaroon.com/article/2021/4/9/covid-advice-long-hauler/

While it felt great to affect change at such a large institution, the best thing to come out of that situation was meeting Rachel. Rachel is a fellow graduate student and long-hauler who contracted the virus around the same time as me. Someone from Student Disabilities Service sent her the article I published in our school paper about Long COVID and she reached out, kickstarting a friendship that has become a lifeline.

She validated my experience, helped me understand what I was going through, and we traded tips and resources that could advance each other's recovery. She is the one who connected me with the Body Politic online support group for COVID long haulers, which has introduced me to so many new long haulers who are experiencing the same things as me. Connecting with this group has made me feel less alone and given me hope in my lowest moments.

Rachel and I are also both campus activists working to make the university more accessible for fellow disabled students in the classroom. Despite being in different programs targeting different administrators, we have supported one another through strategy and solidarity. I honestly do not want to imagine what life would be like if I had never met Rachel, or if I had never connected with the larger long-hauler community.

There have been many moments during this pandemic, and my recovery, where it has felt like every person was out there fighting for themselves (cue flashback to the empty grocery stores of March 2020). In moments like those, it's easy to believe that we are meant to go through all of this on our own. Thanks to people like Rachel and the Body Politic support group, I've come to realize that strength and ease comes not just from our own individual actions, but also by leaning on our community.

# Turn your home into a sanctuary

Falling ill is inevitable, so it's important to live in an environment that doesn't make your condition worse, and where you can gracefully be ill. I have always been a renter. My first Chicago apartment wasn't the best. There was a staircase, which meant that on some days I had to crawl on all fours to get to my room. My landlords were also negligent. When I returned from the emergency room unable to walk, my window blinds had fallen and would constantly wake me up. I asked for a replacement. They took a month and multiple messages to respond.

I was determined to find a better living situation once my lease ended. Finding an apartment was hard. I felt that some landlords looked at me differently when they saw me walk with a cane, and then ghosted me after they learned what I had gone through.

I eventually found an apartment that had an elevator and ramps, was on a bus line, had a dedicated property manager, and a large spacious room with a private bathroom. To top it all off, I would be living with two of my close friends, Brian and Jack. I felt that this place would be a positive environment for me to live in. I decorated my room with lots of motivational messages, pictures of people who mean a lot to me, and filled the air with essential oils.

Although the place has not been completely rainbows and sunshine, I'm a lot happier here. I actually look forward to going home every day, and I can feel good even when I am not feeling my best.

# Find Meaning in Your Suffering

Being a COVID long-hauler sucks. There is no doubt about it. Battling this condition has been the hardest experience of my life. There are days when I feel depressed thinking about all that I've gone through and what I've lost, in terms of time, health, friends, and experiences.

To overcome my despair, I have had to *choose* time and time again to find meaning in my suffering and turn it into something constructive. For me, I've used my experience to think about how to design policies, raise awareness, and mobilize capital and industry to support people with disabilities.

I published an article with Impact Alpha on how impact investors can promote disability justice and support COVID long haulers.[17] My piece went viral and got me an audience with different investment funds who were interested in my ideas. By the end of 2021, I was named by Impact Alpha as one of their Top 10 "Impact Voices" who drove the conversation. [18]

At the University of Chicago, I spoke on mental health panels, supported my classmates through their mental and physical health

---

[17] Rashid, Ibrahim, "Centering disability justice and including Covid long haulers in the post-pandemic economy," Impact Alpha, June 28, 2021. https://impactalpha.com/centering-disability-justice-and-including-covid-long haulers-in-the-post-pandemic-economy/
[18] Impact Alpha, "Impact Alpha's Holiday List No. 2: Ten Impact Voices that drove the conversation in 2021," December 27, 2021. https://impactalpha.com/impact-voices-2021/

challenges, and worked with the University administration to design policies to better support COVID patients and long haulers.

I tailored my degree to understand the systemic drivers that influenced my experience with Long COVID and how policy can be used to support those with less privilege than me. I pursued an independent study exploring how to mobilize capital to invest in the social determinants of health (jobs, food, housing, and health access). I met with fellows at the University of Chicago's Institute of Politics, such as San Juan Mayor Yulin Cruz, and sought their counsel on how to convert pain into power. Mayor Cruz, who led San Juan's response to Hurricane Maria, embodies humility, courage, and hope, and helped me overcome my mental blocks as it related to my own advocacy and the writing of this book.

Finally, I'm working on building my first company, which will produce software to make symptoms manageable for COIVD long haulers. We have already been accepted into different accelerators at the University of Chicago's Business School and through the Clinton Foundation. The depth of my suffering through Long COVID lit the fire in my heart to use every tool at my disposal to make a dent on this issue and provide hope to others.

It's odd to say, but 2021 was both the worst year of my life, and the best. It was the worst because of all the health challenges I faced. But it was also the best because for the first time, I found a purpose.

# Give Yourself Permission to Cry

While I encourage you to find meaning in your suffering and turn it into something positive, I also want to say that this shit sucks, and it's okay to cry. I have cried so much this year. I cried after peeing in a water bottle and spilling urine all over my bed because I could not get up to go to the bathroom.

I cried kicking the snow like a madman because I was frustrated with my brain fog in the middle of finals week. I cried lying in the mud while it was raining because my legs hurt after a swim. I cry when I wake up at night unable to breathe. I cry when I read messages from fellow long haulers in the Body Politic support group. I cry every time I see a homeless person in a wheelchair or with a cane. I've cried when people in my community died from illness, wondering, *will I be next?* And I've cried because every single day is hard. Choosing to show up for yourself every day is so incredibly hard.

In those moments, please be gentle with yourself. You don't have to be high-functioning or accountable to anyone in those moments. All you need to do is show yourself some love, let your negative thoughts dissipate, and take your time to process your emotions. Oh, and tune out the people who are being toxically positive. It doesn't matter how violently you fall; what matters is how gracefully you get back up. Remember to give yourself permission to cry because, frankly speaking, this shit sucks.

## Take Your Mind to Space and Beyond

The pain of this illness can be immense. I learned to cope with it by transporting my mind to space. Seriously. I would go to the place with the asteroids.

I was taught a deep breathing technique by a friend who helped with this. You close your eyes and inhale as deep as you can. First with your stomach and then with your chest. Once you can't breathe in anymore, exhale from your stomach and then with your chest, emptying your body of all air. It's best to do this lying down, but I've done it while sitting up. Do this enough times and you will enter into a deep state of relaxation. Once I was there, I would imagine that I was wearing a spacesuit soaring through the stars and traveling through hyperspace, like the blue hyperspace lanes that Han Solo took the Millennium Falcon through. I soared in and out of those routes, passing distant galaxies, black holes, and the creation of star systems. It was grand. And I would do this almost every time my symptoms flared, or I mourned my lost life. This helped dull the pain.

I learned that if you can close your eyes and silence the world around you, you can imagine a world better than your own that feels real. And once you come back down to Earth, or from wherever you came from, your mind and body might feel just a bit lighter.

## Let Go of Control

When the Omicron variant hit the United States in December 2021, I was terrified. For the first time, I believed that I could actually get sick again. Breakthrough infections were rampant, and I met long haulers in the Body Politic support group who had been reinfected *and* relapsed after believing they were healthy and recovered. I no longer had the confidence that my vaccines and prior infection would protect me and I feared that I was at risk of losing all my hard-won gains. While public health officials encouraged the country to get booster shots, I was reluctant. I felt that the Pfizer vaccine took away my walking.

When the vaccines first rolled out in Spring 2021, I was excited to get it. There was some evidence that vaccines could reduce the severity of the long-haul effects. At that time, I was falling apart, struggling with my new body, and desperate for relief. I scoured social media groups searching for extra vaccines and was one of the thousands to crash county servers when they announced vaccine appointments for my eligibility group. I took polaroid photos of myself getting vaccinated and shared them to Instagram to encourage others to as well. I sang the vaccine's praises to Uber drivers, in long-hauler patient panels, and in articles for my school's newspaper. I was no vaccine skeptic.

However, three weeks after getting my second Pfizer shot, I found myself unable to walk and in the emergency room again. No doctor, let alone those at the Long COVID clinic, ever suggested that my immobility was caused by the vaccine. But I just felt it in my bones that it was. Perhaps this was my way of making sense of the most traumatic moment of my life. It probably was. Regardless, I was terrified to get the booster and swore that I wouldn't, until Omicron emerged and the probability of getting reinfected suddenly increased.

Quickly, I took an antibody test. I was negative. I was vulnerable. Fuck! I could either get the vaccine and potentially risk losing my walking again and develop some other unforeseeable condition. Or I could stay isolated until the "end of the Pandemic"[19] (whenever that would be) and risk getting the virus and relapsing. What was I to do? I decided to get the booster.

I suspected that the vaccine took away my ability to walk, but I knew that the virus made me into a long hauler. I had to make a decision based on what I knew, but it wasn't easy. My heart raced while I waited to get my booster. As the needle pierced my skin, I cried hysterically. The nurse was confused. *What a big baby*, she must have thought.

Getting the booster, I had to accept that I was taking a calculated risk that could backfire. I had to accept that I could not completely control my health and there was a chance of relapse, no matter how hard I tried. I needed to be okay with it. I told myself that if I were to get sick again, heaven forbid, that I would fight it again

---

[19] I hate the phrase "the end of the pandemic." Who is the pandemic actually over for? It's a stupid phrase that is more about politicians and our able-bodied society trying to move on and regain normalcy, than it is about reducing risks for those who are sick and most at-risk.

and win. I had to let go of control and accept the future for whatever it foretold.

## Write Down What You Love about Life

Over the last two years, I learned that you really don't know just how much time  have left, or what will happen tomorrow. Life is precarious and fragile.

At the same time, getting sick reaffirmed to me some of the things that truly mattered. I learned that I love waking up and feeling the sun on my face. I want to spend as much time with my family and immersed in the community as possible. I want to be physically strong and see more of the world. I want to fall in love and feel loved. I want to spend my time doing something beneficial for society.

With whatever time I have left, I am determined to live a life with meaning, and that I can fall in love with. So, I started writing it down. I wrote down everything that I loved about life and looked at it every day. This became my north star and guiding principle that I would work toward every day, bit by bit, no matter how I felt. Slowly over time, I came to realize that I didn't need to have perfect health to experience elements of a good life.

# I'm Still Grieving

At the time of finishing this section, it is March 2022. I just completed my first quarter of full-time graduate school where I did not get sick once or drop a single class. I have started building the endurance to run on a treadmill, achieving a personal best of going twenty minutes before the pain sets in. I have yet to muster the courage to run outside on concrete. I'm trying to build a company, where I'm back to working long days. I have not used my cane since December. It looks like I have recovered and overcome the worst of my long-haul symptoms. All praise be to Allah, Lord of all the worlds. I should be able to look ahead and envision a life free of sickness - but I can't. I am still haunted by the fear of getting the virus again and mourning everything that I lost.

Right now, all of my classmates are either interviewing, searching for jobs, or accepting offers. Despite my recent improvements, I cannot bring myself to look into the future and confidently say what I want my life to look like. It's so hard to go from not knowing whether you're going to have a tomorrow and living life hour by hour to trying to look ahead and plan a career. Yes, I tell people that after I graduate with my master's degree, I either want to work as an investor that focuses on health or climate, *or* I want to run my own startup, *or* I want to do both at the same time.

But in my heart of hearts, I know I just want to rest, above anything else, and soon. Getting Long COVID, finding myself unable to walk, discovering my heart was weaker, losing so many friends, and trying to complete my master's degree has pushed me to my emotional and physical limit. And then some. I am tired. It has only been sixteen months since November 2020, a year and a half since I got sick and started my master's degree. In that time, I feel like I aged a decade.

Some people have looked at me confused when I express my desire for rest, saying I will be happy in the workplace and should get on with my professional life and fulfill my ambitions and potential. I have so much momentum already, they reason. Others are shocked, calling me crazy, when I tell them that I have already turned down jobs in mega-cities all over the world, like London or Chicago.

I hear them, and agree, to an extent. Work is important. It's why I went to graduate school; my career aspirations and desire to help others has given me so much motivation to push myself in my lowest moments. At the same time, I have learned the importance of rest and listening to your body when it tells you that it needs to recharge.

I'm looking forward to finishing my degree and giving myself the space to rest and rediscover myself. This section was my first attempt at processing the events of the last year and a half, but I know there will be more learning on the road ahead.

From a cabin in Kenosha, WI
March 22, 2022

# RELAPSE

# Day 3: March 29, 2022

Over the last two days, my health has spiraled. I am losing my ability to walk, my vision is blurring, and I am having trouble sleeping. Yes, I am reeling from the end of my relationship, but *this* feels like something new. This pain is not *just* heartache. My body is going haywire and out of control, making it impossible to focus on anything but my symptoms. I have to tame my body. But I can't.

None of the tricks in my toolbox are working. Mindfulness, reaching out to friends, sleep aids, eating well, hydrating, CBD oils, using my wearable, electrolytes, vitamins, stretching, progressive muscle relaxation, hot and cold showers, getting sunlight, lying down, eating fruits and vegetables, painkillers, calling a crisis hotline, or reminding myself that I have overcome sickness before and come out of it stronger. None of it is working and I am getting worse.

I'm a runaway train darting towards a cliff with barely enough strength to push down on the breaks. I messaged Terry, saying I was relapsing. He called last night and let me have it. He told me that I should never have stopped seeing him because I only knew the basics of how to stabilize my muscles and nervous system. Because I had settled for "good enough health" and stopped my physical therapy, my body wasn't able to withstand a major stressor like this one. It was only a matter of time before this would have happened, he said. He walked me through a series of exercises to calm my body down. Terry insisted that I see him for the next three weeks and maintain a disciplined physical therapy regimen of three times a day in order to get beyond this relapse. He told me he would come to Chicago personally and beat my ass if I didn't. God bless his soul. I soon went to bed.

Although I only got 4 hours of sleep last night, I woke up this morning feeling okay. I made breakfast and decided to walk to campus. I wanted to test how my legs were doing. There was some pain, but it wasn't bad.

I got to my Management class late and was standing awkwardly by the door. It was my first time using a cane in months and I felt visibly disabled when the instructor called me out and asked me to sit down. It was the first class of the new quarter. The spotlight and attention were unnerving. The professor asked us to introduce ourselves and share an example of a time when we negotiated.

A student who was a Hospital Chaplain told us how over the past weekend, he had to negotiate with the hospital about whether he should encourage a terminally ill patient to accept his impending death or keep on fighting. He wanted him to keep on fighting. I heard that story and started shaking. I saw myself in that patient. Fighting this virus is so hard and sometimes I wonder whether I should keep on fighting, or just give up. I was crying behind my mask and knew immediately that I needed to leave.

I darted out the room and went straight to the Muslim Prayer room. It was locked. Fuck! I took the elevator, went to the highest floor where no one ever goes and made my way to the bathroom. I erupted into tears. I was bawling my eyes out, and the more I cried, the weaker my legs became and the greater the pain. I cried so much that I ended up on the floor and couldn't get up. Here I was, falling apart, on the fourth-floor bathroom of the Harris School of Public Policy at the University of Chicago. Classic.

I immediately dialed Spencer. "Hello, are you okay? What's going on?" He answered. I could barely speak. I was stuttering my words. "Spencer... I ... need... you," I said. My mind was moving at normal speed, but my mouth and tongue were in slow motion. There was a disconnect. "I'm in the bathroom. And... I ... can't... talk... or walk... please come help." He arrived in 10 minutes. As soon as he lifted me up, I fell into his arms crying, and unable to talk. *What was happening to me?*

Another friend of mine came and sat with Spencer and me. We spent the next two hours talking about the symptoms, what it means to be resilient, how the University of Chicago is a pressure cooker, and what it means to be tested by God. Spencer told me he knew how scary it is to lose the ability to speak. He had dealt with it as well.

It was 11 AM, and I had an engineering class at 2 PM. It would be my first-time seeing Yasmeen since we separated. I was scared and nervous. My body was haywire. I made my way to the engineering class. This building was the most inaccessible building I have ever seen, and it was maddening. There were so many stairs and no elevators, and it was poorly marked. My legs throbbed from the stress of trying to find my classroom. I wanted to cry.

When I sat in class, I was exhausted. Yasmeen walked in. When the Professor asked us to introduce ourselves, I tried to speak but I couldn't. "My... name... is... Eh...Brah...heem" I couldn't believe what was happening to me. *Why could I not say my name?* I could barely pay attention in class. I was in so much pain, my head was spinning, my legs were giving out.

I came home at 6 PM. Brian asked how I was doing. Spencer had pulled him aside that morning and told him how my symptoms were relapsing. I was grateful for his support. It reminded me how good of a decision it was to move in with two of my close friends. I spent the rest of the night stretching, talking with family, and trying to stabilize my symptoms. Before I slept, I texted Srishti and Margarita, who were both in Dubai, about what was going on.

# Supporting Another Survivor

*by Katie Schloss*

It was a simple text: "Hey Katie. How's it going?" Even though Ibrahim was technically asking how it was "going" for *me*, I knew—from the formality of it, the way his sentences were punctuated—that for *him*, it wasn't going well.

"Hi! Is everything OK?" But it wasn't. I *knew* it wasn't. And then there it was: "My symptoms relapsed. "Every survivor fears those three words. They are the three words they are afraid of admitting, texting, saying out loud. They are the three words every survivor is afraid of being true. I know this because I am one of them.

Four years ago, I had brain surgery for a three-inch neurocytoma. Half the size of my brain, my neurosurgeon said that he had "never seen a tumor like that before." In asking what he meant by that, my mom figured he meant the size. "No," my surgeon clarified, "I've never seen a tumor like that in someone living before. We usually only see tumors like that in autopsy."

Observing and supporting a friend working through a relapse is a powerless experience; there's nothing anyone can do. The doing and the making—the physical therapy and the appointments and the acupuncture and the healthy eating and the exercises—supporting someone in the actionable to-do list? That's the easy part. The silence and the stillness; how we arrange and rearrange words and sentences over and over again, like Scrabble titles (should we say something reflective or compassionately supportive or…)—all the while worrying: Is this the right thing to say?

In Suleika Jaouad debut memoir, *Between Two Kingdoms*, she writes about what it's like to relapse:

> I begin to think about how porous the border is between the sick and the well… As we live longer and longer, the vast majority of us will travel back and forth across these realms, spending much of our lives somewhere in between. These are the terms of our existence. The idea of striving for some beautiful, perfect state of wellness? It mires us in eternal dissatisfaction, a goal forever out of reach. To be well now is to learn to accept whatever body and mind I currently have.

As I write this, Suleika Jaouad is back in the hospital. This morning when I asked Ibrahim how he was doing, he told me that he was, "falling apart." That his symptoms were "all out of control" and "worse than anything" he had ever experienced.

We talked about what was helping, what was making it worse, how he had found hope in the past, and how he got better last year. "By never giving up, even when all I wanted to do was give up," Ibrahim wrote back. "So, you've done this before," I said. I gave Ibrahim a writing prompt: Write a letter to yourself right now from a place of being healthy. The year is 2030. You've graduated. You're doing well in the world. What would you tell yourself right now? [20]

I wanted Ibrahim to regulate his cortisol levels; to sleep; to eat well. I wanted Ibrahim to imagine himself being healthy again. I wanted Ibrahim to will himself to make that arduous (but inherently worth it) journey back to the Kingdom of the Well once again.

---

[20] Please note, while this one is mine, more writing prompt ideas can be found on Suleika Jaouad's website: https://www.theisolationjournals.com)

# Day 4: March 30, 2022

I woke up at 4 AM with my legs on fire. The hot pain started from my knees and spread to my entire body. I was being engulfed alive. I cried so hard. I struggled to calm my mind and move beyond the pain.

I put on some meditation music and tried to imagine myself in space. My shuttle burst into flames. I listened to some Quranic recitations and begged God to ease my pain. The devil showed up instead. I tried to breathe deeply, but instead of air flowing through my lungs, I felt lava. *Is this the end?*

I checked my phone and saw a message from Margarita and Srishti in our group chat. We hopped on a call immediately, and I told them the pain was too much. Unable to control my tears, I said that I wanted to give up, that I wasn't sure how to keep on living. I was exhausted from fighting, and I wanted to let the fire overwhelm me. I wanted it to burn through my body. I wanted to stop fighting the pain and give into it.

My friends held back their tears, unsure of what to say, but gave me the space to mourn and encouraged me to hold on. I'm so grateful for them. Trauma is what happens when we lack an empathetic witness, as Dr. Jain taught me. They bore witness to my pain and helped me ease my way out.

We stopped talking at 8 AM. Dr. Jain and I had a therapy appointment at 1 PM. During those five hours, I made breakfast without thinking, ate without feeling, and looked out the window without seeing. My body became a vessel devoid of a mind. I sat down, thinking, "I've lived a good life. In twenty-five years, I made wonderful friendships, fell in love, became closer to my family, saw the world, and made a difference in people's lives. If this is the end, then that is okay."

My phone buzzed. It was Rachel, who also has Long COVID. We had not spoken in months. "Hey! I just wanted to check in. How are you doing?" *How did she know?* I told her that I was in the middle of my first relapse, that it was worse than anything I had ever experienced, and I wanted to give up. She told me about her own relapse months prior, shared how it was a common experience, and pointed out how I was managing it better than before. Soon after, Katie messaged as well. As a fellow survivor, she knows what it's like to relapse, and asked how I was able to manage my health last year. She gave me a writing prompt: The year is 2030. You've graduated. You're doing well in the world. What would you tell yourself right now?

1 PM arrived and I finally met with Dr. Jain. I told her how, for the first time, I felt utterly hopeless. That I wasn't sure if I could keep on living like this. That I can't believe *I'm relapsing* after a year of recovery and building resilience. I spent that whole session crying from the pain. We immediately scheduled an appointment for two days later and early next week. Dr. Jain was determined to be there for me and help me hold on. I don't remember what happened over the next few hours. I probably ate lunch and journaled. Spencer called me at 4 PM. He discovered a chiropractor in Chicago who he believed could help me. He also invited me to join him for a meditation group at Rockefeller Chapel in an hour. Touched, I obliged.

Later, I sat with Spencer and the others in silence for thirty minutes, alone with my thoughts. It was a terrifying place to be. I was thinking about the Serenity Prayer. *God grant me the serenity to accept the things I cannot change, the courage to change the things I can, and the wisdom to know the difference.* During the Dharma talk, the facilitator talked about letting go, and just being. He talked about how, if we resist and fight the current, we're going to exhaust ourselves. If we just let ourselves be carried away and feel the water flow through us, we open ourselves to the possibility of finding ease once we reach a destination that we didn't even know existed. He asked us all, what current are we fighting?

I raised my hand. "Hi everyone. My name is Ibrahim, and this is my first time here. I'm fighting a complex medical condition where occasionally, I struggle to walk, speak, see, breathe, and feel. I'm currently experiencing the worst relapse of my life and am fighting so hard to have control and be healthy again. I'm throwing everything in my arsenal at this problem, trying to stabilize my body. But nothing is working. I want to be healthy. But I can't. And I want to give up. I no longer want to fight the pain. I want to stop and let it engulf me. I can't hold on any longer."

I was able to just hold back the tears. The facilitator implored the group to dedicate a minute of silence so everyone could pray for my health. The waterworks burst out at that moment. I came home that night in a daze and sat with my thoughts. I opened my laptop and began writing a letter to myself from 2030.

# Letter from 2030 to the Present

Dear 2022 Ibrahim,

It's me, or you, from the future. I'm your thirty-three-year-old self writing to you because I know you're hurting. Your symptoms are flaring and you're experiencing the worst relapse of your life. You're losing your ability to walk and talk. Your vision is blurring and limbs are freezing. You're struggling to hold on and think straight. Your mind feels disconnected from your body.

Right now, you're trying to grieve the loss of your relationship and battle a host of new symptoms whose intensity and frequency you have never encountered before. You're also unsure whether you will be able to graduate, launch your startup, or maintain your job. You're getting hit on all sides. Your back is up against the wall. Every single coping mechanism you have developed in the last year is rapidly being tested in a short period of time. You feel like you're staring into the abyss, near the point of no return, and don't know whether you can withstand the fire. You're wondering if you should just give into the pain.

Don't. Your life does not end in this moment. It only begins.

I want to give you a glimpse of what the next eight years of your life will look like. First, this moment you are in will pass. You are strong.

This is not the first time life will push you to your absolute limit and it will not be the last. Far from it. You will finish your master's degree. Exactly how long it will take, that's not for me to say. You will build a startup helping other COVID long haulers and publish your book. I won't tell you how your startup or book performs. Somethings are best left as a surprise.

You will learn to live with and manage your health. Notice how I do not say whether you overcome your sickness? You will learn to let yourself fall gracefully, feel your feelings, and gently rise up.

And finally, you will continue to develop your inner peace. You already have a lot of it! Even in this moment, do you not realize how calm you are? Even when you feel like giving up, you are getting through the storm because your body is relying on the habits you cultivated over the last year and your support system is showing up for you. You are fighting with a whole different set of weapons this time around. You're doing such an amazing job. You will plan to tell your newborn child once they are grown about how this is one of the moments where you grabbed life by the horns and yelled, "Come at me!"

You have a lot to look forward to. Hang in there.
2030 Ibrahim

# Excerpt from a Friend's Diary

*by Margarita Louka*

Ibrahim and I met in high school; we've been friends for around eight years. I know of his struggles and journey with Long COVID, and we've actively kept in touch these last few months, despite being separated by distance and time zones. It seemed like he was steadily recovering.

As soon as I woke up and saw my messages, my rest was replaced with bewilderment and dismay. I did not expect to hear from Ibrahim that he was going through a relapse!

After such monumental news, I spent the next few hours in a daze, and was very relieved to get on a video call with him. It is difficult to support a friend when there is so much physical distance between you, but seeing Ibrahim and hearing his voice made me feel like I could offer more concrete support.

My friend was distressed. Hearing him talk about his experience over the last few days with a note of finality to his words was extremely painful, but I tried to stay calm and give him the space he needed to talk. I wanted our friendship to be a safe space where we could both share our pain. The distance between us made me feel powerless; I wished I could do so much more.

We spoke about many things in those few hours, including light-hearted things; they were a good distraction. I could not comprehend exactly what my friend was going through, but I promised myself that I would hold space for him and, despite the distance between us, support him through this.

# Day 5: March 31, 2022

Today, I woke up feeling okay. I spent the morning reflecting on the end of my relationship, writing down all the things that I will miss and cherish about it, the mistakes that I take responsibility for, and what I wish for her. Whether I would ever send my closure letter, I don't know. I went to CVS to buy some fish oil. I was thinking about the book, The Mind-Body Cure, by Dr. Bal Pawa, which goes into the effects of prolonged cortisol exposure in the body. Perhaps my body is having trouble regulating my cortisol? A cursory Google search said fish oil could help with that.

Shortly after, I walked to Regenstein Library to meet my friend, Junaid. I took a week off from work, informing my supervisor that I was relapsing. I wanted to try to get *something, anything* done today. When I stepped into the library, I immediately felt disoriented. From the sounds of people talking to the different hues of lights, every sense was amplified and painful. Junaid looked at me, and by the way he asked how I was doing, I knew he could tell something was wrong.

"I feel like my mind is disconnected from my body." I shared. He asked if I wanted to go to the emergency room. "No. I've gone twice in the last two years," I replied. "No doctor ever knows how to look out for Long haulers. They think it's all in our heads." This was not the last time someone would ask me whether I should go to the ER.

For some reason, leaving the building and standing outside made the sensations go away. We spent the next few hours experimenting by walking in and outside of the building, seeing which spots in the room were triggering my sensations. I would cautiously, slowly move my hands across every surface, turning my head in all directions. People must have thought we were on shrooms. We deduced that the white lights were triggering me. Why, I cannot say. I made a mental note to carry a pair of sunglasses around.

Junaid took me to his place and let me rest in his room. I was too scared of my own body to be alone. I napped for the first time in a week. I woke up, and the sensations were back. Every color I was seeing brought a flash of pain. Rahim came over. I cried in his arms. He's a religious man. I asked if we could pray together. He led the prayer while I sat next to him, arms crossed, bawling to God to ease my suffering. The last time I prayed and cried like this was when my sister was admitted into the ICU during a COVID surge.

I found ease in prayer. It was nice having Rahim next to me. I was struggling to string coherent thoughts in English, let alone recite my prayers in Arabic. Rahim's recitations helped me feel like I was praying too. Prayer helped calm me down. He asked me if I wanted to go to the emergency room. Again, I said no. But I started wondering, should I? *At what point do I just throw in the towel, and go? Should I try to get myself a hospital bed? Should I check myself into a psychiatric ward?*

If none of that works, should I take a leave of absence and move out of Chicago again? The last time this happened, I went to the ER, they told me nothing useful, and I stabilized when I moved out and went to Michigan. *Would I have to do that again?* I would have to completely change my class schedule. One of my professors had rejected my request for a remote learning disability accommodation. *What an asshole,* I thought. *We're living in a pandemic, and people with disabilities should be allowed to participate in school as well.* Without accommodations, moving out would be difficult.

I came home and asked Brian and Jack to meet me in the living room, where I bawled my eyes out. I told them how my symptoms were unbearable, more than anything I had ever encountered. Jack had been my roommate last year. He knew how bad things could get.

I told them how scared I was. I was battling three tidal waves of emotions at the same time. I was mourning the loss of my relationship, I was struggling with my new, unexplained symptoms, and I wasn't sure anymore whether I could complete this degree.

That triple whammy was causing a cycle of stress I could not escape. If I felt okay about my relationship, then the anxiety of new symptoms would set in. If I was able to stabilize my symptoms, my fear of losing my job, startup, and degree would kick in. And then the cycle would repeat itself. I was tormented on all sides. My roommates were empathetic witnesses. I knew that they were at a loss for words. But they held steady and gave me space. They reminded me that I didn't need to make any decisions right now about what to do with my classes or whether to move out. They pointed out how overall I was doing better compared to last year. They helped me sort my thoughts and make a plan for the next day. They pointed out how I was catastrophizing and needed to regain some mental stability by focusing my energy elsewhere. Oh, and they asked me if I wanted to go to the ER. Again, I said no.

After that conversation, I ran a bath with Epsom salts and melatonin, in hopes of inducing sleep and relaxing my muscles. I sat in the dark and meditated for God knows how long. Brian and Jack were right. I was mentally off balance. I was drowning by the currents of my relationship, my future, and my health. I was fighting one wave, while letting the other one knock down my defenses.

A citadel with one wall standing is a citadel that is lost.

## Day 6: April 1, 2022

Throughout the night, I found myself in a dreamlike flow. While battling night terrors, my subconscious rose up to say, "You are strong, defend your citadel!" I would wake up, feel a rush of emotion, but let it pass. In my sleep, I was observing my emotions and letting them be, as opposed to getting carried away by them.

I woke up and the first thing I did was pray. I sat in silence with my thoughts for thirty minutes. "My citadel needs to be strong," I thought. "God, please help me rebuild my walls." I stretched for another thirty minutes, took my supplements, and began to write. (I forgot to eat, which would come to bite me later.)

I had been struggling to decide whether I should check myself into a hospital or not. My symptoms were worse than anything I had ever battled. I caught myself telling people repeatedly throughout the week that I felt like I was on the *verge* of dying (but not *about to*). *At what point would it be best to manage my recovery under the supervision of a doctor?* I thought. I was resistant though.

Today, I spoke to almost every single medical professional and ally in my support system. I called Student Wellness, hoping to reach one of the on-campus doctors who knew me and my condition well. Although he wasn't available to talk, after hearing about my new symptoms, he relayed a message through the nurse to go to urgent care. That advice hit me like a bus. Or a tidal wave. Or an asteroid. My citadel's walls barely held up.

Over the next hour, I sat with my emotions, cried on a bench, and made a series of calls. I first called Ali, my oldest cousin. More than anything, it was nice to talk to my family. I did not want to tell my parents what was going on. Ali reminded me that I *at least* needed to tell them if I was admitted into a hospital overnight. I reluctantly agreed.

The next person I spoke with was Rachel, a fellow Long Hauler. It was a quick call during her break. I told her how frustrated and sad I was. I didn't want to go to the emergency room because I didn't expect the doctors to know what to do with me. I felt like I had met so many doctors whom *I had to educate* about long COVID. She gave me space and said that many with chronic illnesses have that experience. I don't know whether that made me feel comforted or sad. She reminded me that doctors are merely a tool in your arsenal and that I was best equipped to make decisions about my health.

I hopped on the phone with Katie. She told me that if I needed to go to the ER, I should go now. With COVID surges, the wait times would be much longer. Given that it was Friday, she told me, the weekend team would come in around five or six this evening, and they were a lot younger and less experienced. If I was going to mull over this decision, I may as well do it now after starting the clock and increasing my chances of getting the A-Team. She worked at UChicago Medicine and was on standby to sit with me all day in the waiting room, if need be.

I met with Spencer and asked him what to do. He implored me to ignore the people who told me to go to the ER, if they themselves didn't have a chronic illness or know someone who did. They are simply speaking from a place of love and concern and *think* that the emergency room is a place to get better. But it's not. Rather, I should seek the advice and counsel of those who knew that was not always the case.

We walked into the library. My mind started hurting again, the same as the day before. I put on sunglasses and felt much better. We spent the next two hours in our team meeting, discussing feedback on our business model and brainstorming how we could build something that could help COVID Long haulers manage their symptoms. My co-founders had all seen bits and pieces of my relapse over the last week. I took time to share with each of them what I had experienced during the last six days. I wanted them to bear witness to my suffering and *see* the problem that we were trying to solve.

By 1 PM, I spoke with Dr Rasika Karnik, a physician at the University of Chicago Medical Center's Long COVID Clinic. She told me not to go to the emergency room because the doctors there would not know what to do with me. She suggested I seek a prescription for antidepressants to dull the emotions of the last week and hopefully alleviate some of my symptoms.

I called our Behavioral Health line to seek a prescription. They told me that I needed to do an intake first. I begged them to let me skip that process. I already had a therapist for a year and a half. I didn't need to do an intake in four days. I needed something to dull my symptoms right now! The lady on the line kept saying no.

I even yelled, "I'm suicidal!" *I'm not.* I thought it would help speed the process. It didn't. Gah.

I came home and had a meeting with my two internship supervisors. I had taken the last week off because of my relapse. Before I signed on with this new company after leaving IFF in January, I had told everyone on my interview panel that I was a long-hauler and that at some point in my recovery, I could possibly relapse. I had said that for this internship to work for me, they would need to accommodate me in a moment like this. In turn, I had promised them that I would be upfront and transparent about my health status.

I started the meeting by reminding them of that promise and then sharing with them the events of the last week. I didn't even try to hold back my tears. I could tell that they were struggling as well. They promised me that my position would be there when I was ready and able and urged me to focus on my health. I was immensely grateful.

My next call was with Dr. Jain. At this point, I was exhausted. I barely remember what we talked about. I recall telling her about everything that happened on Days 4 and 5 and crying a lot. I asked her what she thought about taking antidepressants. She said that people generally take them if they are resistant to talk-therapy. She didn't believe that I was someone who fell into that bucket. I decided that I would accept a prescription but decide later if I wanted to use it.

79

By now, it was 6 PM, and I realized I had not eaten all day. My body was exhausted and I ate grapes for the next hour in a daze. Tomorrow would be Ramadan, the start of the holiest month in the Islamic Calendar. Rahim and I decided to spend the rest of the night at the local Mosque.

After prayers, I sat in silence with my thoughts. I started thinking about Yasmeen. Throughout the day, I wondered at what point should I tell her how I'm doing. Should I tell her if I go to the emergency room? Should I tell her if I get admitted? At what point do I *need* her? At what point do I *want* her to know? A year ago, she supported me when I first lost my ability to walk, changing the trajectory of my recovery. At this moment, as I grappled with whether to return to the ER, I decided that I would keep her away from my suffering as much as possible.

That's when I realized what love is. Love is deciding to put someone else's needs above your own, even when it is hard. In my lowest moments, I love her more than myself. I love her enough to let her go. I got up, went to the front of the prayer space, put my hands to my face and spoke to God for the first time in years, pleading for mercy.

## Day 7: April 2, 2022

Last night I slept for six and a half hours, the most of the entire week. I woke up feeling sensitive to light and started wearing sunglasses in my room. Today was the first day of Ramadan. *Please God, give me mercy, help me fight this.* Spencer picked me up at 9:45 to take me to the Balancing Center, a chiropractor in the city. The movement of the car, the bumps from the potholes, and the light of the sun were all so painful and disorientating. I was crying the whole way.

Meeting Dr. Ken, the chiropractor, was a profound experience. He had me lie down while holding my legs. He asked me to think about my relationship with Yasmeen before moving my heels. I felt sad and noticed my range of motion shrink. He asked me to think about long COVID, and I erupted into tears, crying hysterically, and my entire body seized up. It was amazing to see the relationship between my mind and body.

He readjusted my spine. He said that the body is like a circuit, where electricity and signals transfer from the brain throughout the body via the nervous system and spine. If the spine is misaligned, it can cause the brain to lose its connection to certain body parts. The body then spends excess subconscious energy trying to compensate for the weakened connection. Thus, when a stressor comes, the body has already used all of its stored energy trying to survive, and the circuit shorts.

This explains why I'm not able to sleep or eat. My body thinks it's being attacked, so it's getting just the amount of sleep needed to get by. As soon as I left Dr. Ken, I felt all the blood and energy in my body flow back to my legs. I felt like I was floating. I was so emotional. I came home and fell asleep for three hours.

When I woke up, I felt like my mind was in a box. I could not recall the names of my friends or family, only their faces. The only thought I could muster was how bad ass Volodymyr Zelensky was and how I hope the Ukrainians kick Putin's ass. *If I ever have a son, I want to name him Amir, short for Volodymyr.* That was the only thought I could muster. I stared at the ceiling for the next two hours. I started to feel cold. I ran a hot bath and sat in the dark. Another two hours passed.

I called Katie shortly after. I told her that I think there is such a thing as too much grit. My mind is too strong. It is holding on despite all of the obstacles it is facing. It is staying centered. But my physical body is weak. There are parts of me that are structurally broken. By being too strong, I asked, am I at risk of ignoring my body even when it is telling me that it is unwell? In my recovery, I've always tried to use my mind to rise above my pain. I thought I understood the two-way street between the Mind and the Body connection, but I didn't. Dr. Ken helped me realize that I needed healing. No amount of mental fortitude could dramatically alter the fact that parts of my inner structure were off.

I told Katie that I'm starting to disassociate my mind from my body. I told her that I was scared of holding on, because it could mean ignoring the needs of my body and make myself worse. Katie encouraged me to make a pros and cons list of why I should keep holding on and rearranged my statements into a balanced thought. Here's what I wrote:

> *Even though continuing to push may make my health worse in the short-term and finding out that my mind doesn't have more control than it does is extremely difficult, it's worth it to continue pushing, because I want to be healthy; I want to be with people I care about (like friends and family); I want to see color; I want to have kids and a family; I want to publish*

*my book, and I want to graduate—all of which can't do unless I continue to push.*[21]

---

[21] I should mention probably here that Katie is training to be a therapist and wants to open her own practice where she coaches entrepreneurs and people with chronic illnesses.

# Letter from 2035 to the Present

Dear Ibrahim,

It's your thirty-eight-year-old self, writing to you. I know you spoke with thirty-three-year-old you just a few days ago. I'm sorry that I wasn't available. We're currently juggling baby number two right now. I know that you are struggling. I remember what it was like to be in your shoes. Please don't give up. Keep holding on.

You just left the emergency room for the third time in less than two years, and they told you that you were perfectly healthy, that they could not figure out what was wrong, and sent you home - again. They told you that there was honestly nothing they could do for you, and you just had to keep holding on. The only thing they could give you was medication to sleep better.

Right now you're sitting in the dark, in your bathtub crying into the water, wondering if this life is worth it. You're begging God to give you ease. Begging for his forgiveness. Begging for mercy.

I need you to please hold on. I need you to keep fighting. I need you to meet your future wife, who is going to love you unconditionally, irrespective of how sick or healthy you are. I need you to hold your first child, your beautiful daughter, in your arms, and experience a new father's love. I need you to watch the birth of your son. I need you to keep fighting. You have a future to look forward to.

You also have a present that is worth fighting for. In this moment, you are seeing friends show up for you in every way possible, and your life is magically different compared to last year. Today, you came home from the emergency room and instead of crying alone in your bedroom, watching Netflix and eating McDonalds, you had Catherine and Katie by your side. Katie was with you almost all day in the ER, waiting with you. She brought you food, and helped you advocate for yourself with the nurses. You have Catherine, who sat with you in the hospital, held you when you cried, and gave you flowers. You came home, and Rahim, Junaid, Jack, and many others were there. They gave you hugs, held space with you, and left you cards. Briana, who hardly ever shows emotion, almost cried while on the phone with you earlier in the day. You are not alone. You have friends who care about and love you.

You are growing up, and becoming a better man, even if you feel like mush right now. You also advocated for yourself so well today! You spoke about the biology of your condition and demanded certain tests. You called out nurses for giving you tests that you didn't need. You recognized staff when they were empathetic and told them how much you appreciated them. One nurse even said to you, "I never even knew what Long COVID was until this moment." You are one hell of a fighter.

Now, please, get up. Get up Ibrahim. Get up. Don't give up. Keep holding on. You're doing great. Even though you feel alone, you need to imagine yourself as Rey from the Rise of Skywalker, who is facing down Emperor Palpatine on Exegol with a legion of fallen Jedi behind her. Instead of the Jedi Knights, behind you are all of your friends and family who care about you. They're all right by you, watching over you. Please do not give up hope. You can and will fight this. I have faith in you.

Sincerely,
2035 Ibrahim

# Supporting a Friend from Afar

*by Briana Lopez*

I first met Ibrahim during our senior year of college. He was bright, intelligent, adventurous, and always the jokester. Our conversations revolved around world politics and strategizing our post-graduate careers. After graduation, our friendship grew as we both cut our teeth amidst the demands of working in foreign aid in Washington, D.C., and when he later moved to Chicago for graduate school.

I received a phone call from him on April 3, 2022. I knew he was relapsing, so I was not surprised to see a call that afternoon. From the moment we started talking, I could tell that something was different. His tone was off, different, yet still calm and at ease. After some light banter, I asked what he was doing and he replied, "I'm just hanging out at the ER."

"I don't think people just *hang out* at the ER," I said. Shortly after, the topic of a final goodbye was raised. It was unexpected, but I managed to muster out words that I believe were helpful at the time. Although, looking back at it now, it may have been just a hodgepodge of thoughts. How exactly do you support a close friend who is sick and facing such stressful realities from so far away? How do you convey a meaningful message to help them in their time of need? After he said his farewell and thanked me for our friendship, I could sense he wanted a bit of a distraction from reality, so I opted to tell him more about my life. The remainder of our conversation felt like any other, and I was glad that even at wit's end, we managed to make the most of it. At one point I asked if he was at peace, and he replied that he was.

The truth is, I was not ready to lose one of my best friends. I understood, though, that it wasn't my choice whether someone left this world or not. That bright, intelligent and adventurous jokester was still there, but he was tired. Exhausted. I knew he was strong enough to keep going, but damn it was tough.

To support a friend through so much pain is to acknowledge that the exhaustion is there, but to hope that their will to continue living is even bigger.

# Day 8: April 3, 2022

There was a knock on the door. I came out of my meditation. "Come in," I said. The doctor walked in. "We've run through all of your labs, and you look perfectly fine. You are one of the healthiest twenty-five-year-olds we have ever seen, and that's saying a lot. We see nothing wrong with your muscles or nerves that should explain why you are unable to walk, or any of your other symptoms.

Our behavioral insights team recommends that you continue to see your psychologist, since you have already developed many of the coping skills needed to withstand a condition like yours. We're unsure why you are unable to sleep. You're already doing everything from a behavioral perspective that we would recommend to optimize and improve your sleep. The best we can do is prescribe you Xanax. This doesn't mean that what you are feeling is not real, but we are unable to see or do anything. We're going to recommend that you be discharged and go home."

And there it was. My third emergency room visit ended the same way it always does. *With nothing.* Nothing but a Xanax prescription and being told to keep holding on, keep doing everything I was already doing, keep fighting. I sat in silence in that small room with the white fluorescent light for the next hour. Catherine walked in. She had flowers. She gave me a tight hug. I tried to force myself to smile, but I couldn't. I whimpered and she held me close.

"Is it wrong that I wanted them to admit me tonight? That I wanted them to believe that my body was actually failing me?" I asked her, or God. I wasn't sure who I was talking to at that moment.

This whole week I felt like I was on the *verge of death*, staring at my last moments, and every system in my body was pumping with adrenaline, trying to keep me alive. When I woke up this morning, I found myself writing a farewell letter. Writing this book is one of the few things allowing me to cope and give me meaning amidst all this sensory loss, and I wanted to make sure that it sees the light of day. I shared the original manuscript with some of my close friends and gave explicit instructions on how I would like it to be published and shared with my loved ones if I was not around.

Katie asked if I was thinking about taking my own life and I said no. I said I was accepting my body's limitations. She pointed out how final farewells are signs of suicide. I could feel myself giving up. This morning, I made the painful decision to go to the emergency room. The last time I'd gone, I waited for twelve hours with nothing to eat. This time I packed food, books, headphones, my laptop, and messages of encouragement and hope received over the months and years. I made sure to clean my room and ask my friends to have flowers ready for me when I came home. At some point, I knew I would come home, and probably feel really depressed. I needed a way to soften the blow.

At the emergency room, I painstakingly told every doctor what was going on. I walked through every symptom and feeling I experienced over the past week. I told them how I wasn't making this up and how this was a last resort for me. I said how I spoke with every single clinician in my support system and after careful deliberation, felt I needed to be here. I told them that I did not expect them to cure me of Long COVID. No one could. All I needed was some relief. I wasn't able to sleep. I was losing my ability to swallow. The adrenaline pumping through my veins was destroying me. I needed something to stabilize me. I could feel the next wave of adrenaline coming and was not sure if my body could withstand another week tethering by the abyss.

So, when they told me that there was nothing they could do, I felt defeated. I wanted someone to tell me that my symptoms were real enough to warrant attention, that the pain I was feeling was not in my head, but it was biologically, medically present in my body. That there was *something* that could be done, that there was some intervention that could stabilize me. There wasn't.

I asked myself the same question that every long hauler faces at some point. *Is this all in my head? Am I making this up? Am I going crazy?* For the first time, I wasn't sure.

## Day 9: April 4, 2022

I woke up this morning angry. My thoughts were racing. *I can't believe I went to the emergency room last night.* The night before, one doctor came in and told me I was fine and ready to be discharged. A moment later, a nurse said I was to be transferred to a different hospital into a psychiatric ward. I demanded an explanation for the inconsistency. She never came back to correct her mistake or apologize. I chewed out the nurse who reaffirmed that I was, in fact, ready to be discharged, even if I knew it wasn't her fault. *The system is broken.*

I could feel myself getting angry at everything around me. Every thought I had was muffled in a blinding rage. I knew the anger would make my symptoms worse, make my head hurt, weigh me down, and so on. I didn't care. I didn't try to control myself for once. *I deserve this pain. The only thing that makes sense right now to me is that I am in pain. Even if no one is going to believe me, I can at least have clarity that my suffering is real.*

I needed to get food in me. I was still having difficulty swallowing. The sun was out and I walked to Trader Joes to buy yogurt, soup, smoothies and bananas. I needed to keep feeding myself. I needed to tell my body that it was okay even if it was not. I needed to eat. It was a nice day. The sun was warm (for Chicago's standards). I was still pissed off, but slightly less. I loved the sun.

I came home, reread the last few chapters of this book, and realized I was actually making progress. I was holding on. I tried to change my perspective on the ER. They said my body was exceptionally healthy. Everything I was doing was stabilizing myself. I was holding it together. For the longest time, relapsing and going to the emergency room were two of my biggest fears and sources of trauma that stopped me from fully participating in my life. I just went to the emergency room and back and… it wasn't too bad. I had snacks, after all. My citadel's walls had crumbled. I needed to shore them up.

I sat in my chair and meditated. In the past, I would say to myself, "My wall that is protecting me from sadness over my health or future is broken, I need to rebuild this wall." This time, I didn't specify any particular meditation. All of my walls had fallen. I just sat for what felt like an hour imagining all four walls of my citadel being rebuilt, without any specific attention as to which.

I thought about Yasmeen. Something in my heart told me that I should reach out to her and let her know that I was okay. She didn't know I had been in the emergency room yesterday. I kept that news tightly held and only within a select circle of friends. *Maybe I'll message her tonight.* I got up. I picked up my phone.

One missed call and text from her. Two minutes ago. *What?*

I called her immediately. She sounded distressed. She told me how she had had this feeling that I was not okay. She said she had been fighting the urge to stop by my apartment, to check in on me, but hadn't. I asked her if she wanted to know what had happened, she said yes, and I told her about the last twenty-four hours.

Early in our relationship, she wrote me a letter saying, "You're a strong and capable man, and I'll always be right beside you." I told her how that note was one of the few things I took with me into the ER. I told her that I was holding on, had a lot of doctor appointments lined up this week, and that I wanted her to focus on herself.

Later that evening, I received a message from a classmate. Apparently, her partner was experiencing all sorts of symptoms, including an inability to move his arms, tingling, and numbness. They were getting ready to go to the ER.

I spoke to him as calmly as I could, channeling my inner Katie. I told him that he should consider the mental toll of going to the ER. It was 6 PM. If he went now, he might come back at midnight. He might be told just to go home and rest. The emergency room itself is a traumatic place. He needs to shore up his mind for the journey, the stay, and the return. This moment can be traumatic, but what he does *now* will determine how hard that blow will land.

I told him and his partner the importance of controlling the mind. How thoughts could induce paralysis. I asked him about his general lifestyle. He hadn't been sleeping or eating well the last few weeks. The stress of the University of Chicago was getting to him (God, I know that feeling). I asked him if he had eaten, he said no. I asked him if he thought he was dying. He said no, just that his arm was numb. I asked him if he could hold on for a few more days. He said yes. I said that it would be worthwhile for him to take some time to calm the mind and body down, that he was likely experiencing an intense fight or flight response, that he should try to manage his symptoms, and rebuild the citadel in his mind, so that when he does go to the ER, if he chooses to make that decision, he will be able to emotionally withstand it. I asked him to imagine the year was 2030. His older self was writing a letter to himself today. What would it say?

I told him that I have dealt with similar muscle tension and sudden loss of sensations. He asked me if he should keep pushing, if he should keep fighting with his arm. I told him no. I told him he cannot disassociate himself from his body, that he needs to love it, and that there is an impermanence to life and health. We will never fully be in the kingdom of the well or the kingdom of the sick. We will always be living in between and he needs to find acceptance in that. I could feel him calming down. Katie would be so proud if she could hear me.

He asked me what to do. I told him that warm baths help with blood flow. I suggested he take a bath in Epsom salts. It was good for the mind and good for the body. He agreed. His partner came on the line, saying that he was calming down. I asked her how she was doing. She put on a strong face. I told her that she must be feeling powerless at this moment. I told her that when we suffer, we never suffer alone. Even if it is the sick person in pain, the people around us go on this journey with us.

I told her that even though she doesn't know what to do, by holding steady and giving space to her partner, she would be able to support him. I encouraged the guy to ask her after our call how she feels about this moment, to be vulnerable and talk about this moment of fear and powerlessness. Although these conversations are painful and emotional, and in these moments we're most likely to put up walls, I said that it was a beautiful, intimate, and powerful experience to acknowledge fear together and declare that we're going to get through it. I told him that as soon as he recovers, he better love his partner extra hard to show gratitude for supporting him.

They asked me how I learned all of this, and I said how Yasmeen had been my rock in every single moment of my illness. Even though she always felt powerless when I fell ill, her presence carried me through it. They told me I was lucky to have her, and I agreed.

## Day 10: April 5, 2022

Today, I got out of bed, took a warm shower, loaded up on my supplements and vitamins, spread CBD around my body, hydrated, meditated, prayed, stretched, made a smoothie, packed a box full of liquid food, got dressed, wore my sunglasses, put on my knee braces, wore my favorite *Captain America* T-Shirt, opened a *Spotify* playlist of all the Power Rangers' theme songs, grabbed my cane, and made my way to the bus stop.

The bus was full and no one was giving space for me. I put my cane in the air and asked loudly, "Can someone make space for me to get to the priority seating?" No one answered. "Come on, don't be a fucking ass hole. Move!" I used to be really timid in demanding my right to space. Not anymore.

I got to my Management class, the same one with the hospital chaplain. The same one whose professor rejected my disability accommodations. During the ten-minute break, I approached him directly and introduced myself. I told him that I would like him to approve my disability accommodation, and shared that I just came out of the hospital after fighting for my life all of last week. I told him that I would be the hardest working student in his class because I'm fighting for my life and my ability to access my education. I said that I needed him to approve my accommodation. I had every intention of showing up to every single class, but if I had to go back to the hospital, then I wanted to continue learning the content *at least* remotely. He conceded and said he would approve it.

It amazed me to think that if someone fell sick and was hospitalized, the University would accommodate them at that moment. But if someone with a disability proactively says that it is *possible* they will need an accommodation *in the future,* it's perceived as asking for "special permission" and preferential treatment. We're not asking for special treatment, rather we're acknowledging that the future is unpredictable, and we know ourselves well enough to give a heads up.

I went from class to meet with David Chrisinger. I just wanted to chat with one of the few staff at the University whom I truly considered a mentor and a friend. Soon after, I had an intake with a psychiatrist. Dr. Karnik suggested that I seek a prescription for antidepressants and the emergency room gave me Xanax. I have a strong aversion to medication, out of fear of the side effects. I wanted guidance on how to make an informed decision about drugs. I was running late for class. I knew Yasmeen would be worried if she didn't see me. En route, Terry messaged me saying he would have to cancel our appointment scheduled right after class, freeing up my evening.

I walked into class 10 minutes late. During the break, Yasmeen gave me the tightest hug of my life. I was relapsing all of class, feeling adrenaline rise and fall in my body. The fluorescent light was blinding and my body was burning, on and off, on and off, on and off. I stepped out to run my arms under hot water to stimulate blood flow. I applied CBD oils to my neck. I massaged myself. I don't even know what we discussed in class, to be honest. The professor approached me after his lecture and affirmed that he was committed to helping me stay in the class and would provide all the accommodations needed to help me succeed. I was so immensely grateful. *This* is what it should be like.

I got home, sat in my bathtub, stretched, and then made my way for Iftar, the time at sunset when Muslims break their day long fasts during the holy month of Ramadan.

# Day 11: April 6, 2022

This morning I felt like mush. I woke up but could not get out of bed. I was tired. So incredibly tired. The day before really took a toll. My body was drifting in and out of sleep. I got out of bed at 9 AM, the latest I left my bed since the start of my relapse. I started organizing my room. It was a total mess. I took my supplements, made sure to hydrate, stretch, meditate, and pray. My body was on autopilot. My mind was so tired. It was nice to put it to sleep while I let the body do its own thing for a bit.

Exhausted, I lay down in bed at 12:30. *I never finished the closure letter that I wrote for Yasmeen*, I thought. I opened it and added a few things here and there until my therapy appointment with Dr. Jain. I told her everything that had happened since last Friday and how I went to the ER. I told her that I was struggling to believe that I was still sane. The experience of going into the emergency room made me feel like I was losing my mind, questioning whether my symptoms were real. Those thoughts were unsettling.

Our appointment ended at 2 PM and I had to make my way downtown to see Dr. Ken. Once I settled in, he had me lay on my back while adjusting my legs. He asked me to think about a series of thoughts: betrayal, the emergency room, walking, the end of my relationship, feeling calm, hope, and so on. With each thought, he would adjust my legs, pushing on them, trying to restore mobility. I asked him why he wanted me to imagine certain thoughts. He said it was because I am not just a COVID long-hauler. I am a person with feelings and emotions. Those emotions were creating tension in my body that were restricting my range of motion. He was training my body to no longer lose mobility when it felt a certain way. He was helping my body unlearn its own trauma. He was treating me as a person, not just a sickness.

When I walked out of that appointment, my legs felt like slime. I went for a walk around downtown, just seeing where the wind would take me. I saw a FedEx store. *Should I print this closure letter for Yasmeen?* Something inside me said I should. I sat in a Starbucks, made a few edits on my phone, before going to FedEx. Just as I printed the document, stapled it together, and held it in my hand for the first time, my phone rang. It was Yasmeen.

"Hello? Are you okay?" she asked. "Yes… why would I not be?" I was confused and shocked at her call. "Are you sure? What are you doing right now?" "Um, I just came out of a doctor's appointment." It was true. I didn't want to tell her exactly what I was doing, as I held her letter in my hand. "Well, I just had this feeling that either you were in serious trouble or you were manifesting me. You need to stop manifesting me. It's exhausting! So, I just had to call to figure out what's going on."

"Well, um, if you must know . . . I'm at FedEx downtown printing a closure letter for you. I was thinking about sticking it on the front of your door." "Oh my God, you're downtown? You're writing me a letter? Why would you stick it on my door instead of giving it to me directly!" "Because I'm trying to respect your desire for space!"

We laughed hysterically. We were in disbelief. I came over shortly after, setting foot in her apartment for the first time since the day we separated. I sat with her while she read my letter, going through fourteen pages of all the things I would miss, cherish, take responsibility for, and what I wish for her. It was a sweet, somber, and loving moment.

## Day 12: April 7, 2022

Today I still felt like mush. But a bit better. Last night was emotionally surreal. I spent the morning cleaning my apartment (again), doing my self-care routine, and trying, for the first time, to get *some work* done this week.

I returned to Dr. Ken, my chiropractor. I told him how, after our session yesterday, I felt like my body was no longer on fire and that somehow I found the clarity and courage to finish my letter for Yasmeen, which resulted in us talking honestly for the first time. I told him how cathartic it was. I strongly believe that the pain in my body from long COVID was stopping me from being the best version of myself and showing up in my relationship.

During our session, my mind drifted back to Yasmeen. She gave me a lot of motivation to keep fighting and holding on. Last night, I told her how absolutely exhausted I was. Last week, I felt like a runaway train, verging towards the edge of a cliff. Going to the emergency room was me falling to the bottom. In a way, being on the train was comforting. There was a clarity of purpose. *Survival.* Now that I had fallen, and my symptoms had somewhat stabilized, the challenge was getting back up. My tank was empty and I was exhausted. This felt like a slow burn that was even harder to shake off.

There was a moment last night where I was lying on Yasmeen's couch, unresponsive. I was absolutely exhausted. I knew she was there and talking to me. I knew where I was, but I couldn't bring myself to speak. I had been looking at my body from the outside in, trying to yell at myself to get up and speak, but I couldn't. Yasmeen had been worried. Through tears, she had told me that she needed me. She needed me to keep holding on and to keep fighting, and she needed me in her life. She told me that she loved me. And there it was. A flicker in my brain.

Hearing her say that she needed me switched the lights back on, reminding me that I needed to keep fighting. I can do that by not giving up, by doing all these appointments, by working on getting better, by working on being better. By becoming a healthier man and a better man. By surviving. By living. By finding acceptance in where I am, rather than where I want to be. By not letting the pain of the past hold me back, or optimism about the future recklessly propel me forward. By accepting that I'm neither sick nor healthy. I am somewhere in between and can learn to move forward. I will move forward. For myself. For her. For my family. I came home at night and sat in my bathtub for another two hours. It's in the silence between moments where we find God, hope, and love.

# RECOVERY

# Day 1: April 10, 2022

I am exhausted. But I'm still here, and I'm calm. I no longer feel like I am relapsing. You know how Robert F. Kennedy wrote *Thirteen Days*, his memoir of the Cuban Missile Crisis? I could probably write a book titled *Twelve Days: My Journey from the Brink of Long COVID*. What a fucking ride.

I'm trying to pick myself up now and rebuild. My relapse began before the first day of the spring quarter here at the University of Chicago. I never even looked at my syllabi, organized my calendar, or did any of the readings. I basically missed the first two weeks of school. God, I hate having to play catch up. I've been here before, and I know I'll be able to pull myself up. Last year, I got horribly sick in the spring and had to move out. It was a traumatic experience that I'm still reeling from. This time around, I'm hoping to better process my emotions, and experience a bit more post-traumatic growth as opposed to post-traumatic stress.

First things first, I want to be a better partner to Yasmeen. Without realizing it, I had a fixed mindset as it related to my health. I was absolutely terrified of getting sick again and relapsing that I did *everything* in my power to avoid even the *probability* of sickness or COVID exposure. If I felt that my WHOOP stats were on the *verge* of falling, I would go into survival mode, reschedule my day, and become a semi-functioning shell. This mental exhaustion meant that I was too damn burned out to be present for her, let alone myself. I need to work on improving my health. Going to the chiropractor and maintaining my appointments with Dr. Jain and Terry would help. But most importantly, I need to learn to just *let it be*. I cannot be so scared of the possibility of sickness that it holds me back from experiencing the joys of life. I need to live!

Second, I want to be kinder to those around me. We never suffer alone. There is an army of people around me who have witnessed my suffering and felt pain alongside me. They have moved Heaven and Earth for me and filled my cup even when theirs were empty. I need to make it a point to look out for them and show my gratitude and appreciation.

## Day 4: April 13, 2022

I'm fighting on five fronts right now. I'm still processing the fact that I spent the last few weeks watching my health rapidly deteriorate. No one seems to understand the severity of what this relapse felt like. The fear, the pain, the confusion. Not my family, not my friends, not even myself. People have told me that I am overreacting and just need to chill out. Fuck them. I'm retraumatizing myself by remembering the experience, in the most mundane of moments.

I'm trying to learn to love Yasmeen differently. Because of my symptoms, I didn't allow myself to be present or intentional. Every couple has "that one big fight" over a "little thing." I'm trying to rewire myself to address that. It's hard work. It's really, really hard. I think it's worth it, because she's worth it, but it's hard, nonetheless.

I'm still fighting my symptoms. I'm jumping from doctor appointment to doctor appointment. I'm either at a chiropractor, with my therapist, getting blood work done, seeing a psychiatrist, talking to insurance, and so on. If I'm not doing that, then most of my free moments are spent meditating, stretching, trying to reset my nervous system, taking supplements, forcing myself to eat well, hydrating, sitting (and crying) in a bathtub, and so on.

I'm trying to build a startup to help COVID long haulers. We presented earlier this week at a summit hosted by the Clinton Foundation. We received such overwhelmingly positive feedback. In every audience we are in, there is someone who is or knows a COVID long-hauler. The work we're doing is important and wide reaching. It's also really emotionally draining. I once called a crisis hotline in the midst of my relapse and told them how scared and frustrated I was by Long COVID. They told me that I must believe that there are people working on the problem trying to bring relief to folks like me. I paused and told the guy that I'm one of those people trying to build something for Long COVID, and I don't believe in myself. He didn't really have anything to say to that.

Finally, I'm trying to just get by in my graduate courses. Yesterday we did a simulation for our Management class. My team set a class record. It feels good to do well in school, even if I'm barely present. These are the five walls of my citadel. When one is weak, the other ones fall. I'm on a tightrope, trying to balance and hold on. I'm on the edge, dangling, staring at the abyss.

I envy those who don't spend every waking moment fighting for their health. Truly. I wouldn't wish this experience on anyone, even though it's taught me a lot of hard-earned wisdom. I know in a way that it's a blessing. I'm twenty-five years old, and most people my age do not experience a health crisis or grapple with their mortality like this. It's something they will develop as they age into their 30s, 40s, and 50s, or later.

Our bodies are temporary vessels of health, and we're all just on the verge of becoming disabled someday. I just happen to be someone who has experienced this earlier in life. That's why I feel so alone. I know the silver lining is that, God willing, I will get to experience more years of life with this hard-earned wisdom. I will get to walk this Earth longer than most, having tasted illness and suffering, known the depth of my own despair, and risen up. I will have become more gentle, more appreciative, take things less for granted, and so on. I know this is the silver lining. It just sucks so much right now.

## Day 19: April 28, 2022

It's been just over a month since the start of my relapse. Today, I exercised for the first time since mid-March. I went for a swim. Water is my place of peace and healing. Submerged, my body felt different. I tried to swim. I was weaker; I was slower. Twenty minutes in and I felt like I got hit by a bus. *I guess that's it for today.*

I got out of the pool and went to the locker room. I undressed and weighed myself. I was a few pounds lighter than before. I looked at myself in the mirror. I could see the impact that my sickness had on me.

## Day 27: May 6, 2022

One year ago today, I found myself underneath a tree, reading a book, and unable to get up. I fell. I tried again. My legs were weak. I could barely walk. I went to the emergency room. They didn't know what was going on. They told me to go home and rest. I would soon drop my graduate classes and move to Michigan to live with my aunt, kickstarting my whole 'Long COVID' journey, and the foundation of this book.

Today, I'm battling my second COVID Infection. I've not gotten tested. I don't want to deal with the trauma of seeing another positive result. But I've been running a fever this whole week and people around me are getting sick.

I'm putting two and two together and assuming I have it, and it sucks. My new internship also just informed me that I was fired. *What assholes.*

## Day 39: May 18, 2022

I am so tired. I stopped quarantining early last week, but before I could catch a breather, I had to go full steam ahead refining my startup's pitch. This past Monday was the second round of the Social New Venture Challenge accelerator that I'm competing in. It was exhausting. But we did it. We'll find out in a week if we're going to the finals where we will compete for $175K in funding.

A lot of people believe in me, and my company's idea. Many have told us that even if we don't place as a finalist or win this competition, we should keep working on the idea. At the same time, I'm struggling to see myself as an entrepreneur. I'm just some kid who got sick and had an idea. I don't even know what a pivot table is in Excel. I'm also scared. If I'm a founder of an early-stage startup, how am I going to provide myself health insurance? If I build a long-COVID focused company, am I outing my disability to the world? Especially after my last employer pulled the plug on me when I got sick, I'm *really* struggling to be confident and proud of myself, and see my sickness as a strength, rather than a weakness. My self-esteem has definitely taken a beating.

I'm really, really tired. This quarter has been so much. From my relapse to the end of my relationship, to rebuilding it, to getting COVID again, to starting a whole new treatment plan, to trying to manage my health, to building my company, to losing out on a job that I was really excited for, to being on the verge of *graduating* and planning my future. I've taken a lot of hits, and I am very, very tired. I'm so tired that it's hard to be excited about the fact that Yasmeen and I are back together. I'm looking forward to taking a break. Honestly, I could use it.

## Day 47: May 26, 2022

We didn't make the cut. We're not going to the finals for the Social New Venture Challenge. *Damnit!*

## Day 50: May 29, 2022

Yesterday was the first time that I played. I was in a lot of pain when I woke up in the morning, so I had to hunker down to manage myself. It was frustrating. I told myself to do yoga, I told myself to meditate, to stretch, to do all of the different self-care bullshit I have learned over the last two years when I feel down, but I just couldn't bring myself to do it.

Instead, I lay in bed and let the time go by as I read comic books. It was awesome. I then went to my living room to play Star Wars Battlefront on my Xbox One. That night, I surprised Yasmeen by buying a bunch of toy guns that sprayed bubbles, a frisbee, and playdough. *This is what we are going to do today!*

We spent the evening acting like toddlers in the park, with our bubbles, before coming home to make dinosaurs with playdough. Ever since I got Long COVID, I stopped playing. Whatever free time I have has been spent trying to manage my health, stabilize my symptoms or exercise. And then it's back to work. I make very little time for play. I want to change that.

## Day 63: June 11, 2022

I had my graduation ceremony last weekend. My parents, sister, uncle, and cousins all flew down to Chicago to see me. Even though I didn't "officially" graduate, since I still have two classes to go, it felt amazing to walk across that stage.

I sat with Spencer and we both acknowledged how there were so many moments in the last few years where we both doubted whether we would ever experience this moment. Our health was so tenuous. But it happened. And it was grand.

Now I'm in California, staying with my mom and sister. I landed two days ago on Wednesday and since then, I had my first post-grad job interview, spent the day at a theme park, and an investor reached out wanting to learn more about my company.

I also caught up with my old college roommate, Ali Al-Haj and his girlfriend, Mary, and we hiked a mountain. It took us three hours to reach the top. We were above the clouds, saw a helicopter and airplane fly right by, and watched the sunset across the Los Angeles skyline. I looked at my watch; I burned a thousand calories on the way up. My legs were sore, but not the type of pain that meant I had to slow down, breathe, and pull my cane out. No, it was the pain of pushing my body, hiking up a mountain, and making it to the top. It felt good. I felt good.

## Day 177: October 3, 2022

A lot has changed in the last four months. When I was in California in June, I interviewed for a job in finance and sustainability that I would later accept.

I returned to Chicago in July, started working part-time while I wrapped up my last two classes of my graduate degree. After spending a lot of time at the Balancing Center with Dr. Ken, I decided to challenge myself to start running again. By early August, I competed in my first 5K race. That was one of the best days of my life.

A few weeks later, I moved into a new apartment with my cousin from Pakistan. The Clinton Foundation reached out, inviting my team to present our startup alongside Chelsea Clinton in New York. Afterwards, I traveled to Costa Rica for a much-needed two-week vacation. There, I lounged on the beach, learned how to surf, hiked a mountain, drove an electric scooter around a volcano, danced, ate new food, spent time in nature, cried in the rainforest, and gave myself a lot of space to work through my emotions.

My takeaway after all of this? My life did not end with my sickness. It only began. I spent two years going slow, learning how to walk and live again. Now it's time to move forward. Without fear. With hope.

# Acknowledgments

There are so many people to thank for a project like this. The first thank you goes to my family, my mom Fauzia, my dad Rashid, and my 'baby sister' Eesha—all of whom have given me enough love and support to last a lifetime.[22] You all are the best family I could ever ask for.

Thank you to Yasmeen for being my rock. Thank you to Spencer Gudewill for teaching me that the "Obstacle is the Way," and clearing so many paths for me. I wouldn't be where I am without you. Thank you, Katie Schloss, for being a wonderful mentor and friend, guiding me out of the abyss.

Thank you to Nausheen Rafi and your baby Musa for giving me a loving place to stay when I was unwell. Thank you to Rachel for reminding me that I'm not alone. Thank you to David Michael Chrisinger for being my mentor, professor, editor, and friend. You helped me become a better trauma-informed writer who could transform his own pain into something meaningful.

Thank you to Dr. Divya Jain, Dr. Terry Moore, and Dr. Kenneth Bennet, Dr. Jerome Wilczynski, and Dr. Rasika Karnik for helping me regain my abilities and adopt a "growth mindset" as it related to my health. You have all been so incredibly instrumental in my recovery.

---

[22] Eesha is actually older than me. But I try not to think about it too much.

Thank you to my amazing supervisors, Krissy Pelletier, Timothy Docking, Yi Wei, and Jose Cerda III, who invested in my professional development despite my challenges. Thanks to my academic support staff at the University of Chicago, including Hanna Seferos, Eman Alsamara, and Kate Biddle, for advocating for me relentlessly so that I could finish this degree.

Thank you to my company's advisors and supporters, Lenka Beranova, Kaakpema 'KP' Yalpaalam, Ryan Prior, Tara Cunningham, Nathan Pelzer, Myeashea Alexander, Ragina Arrington, Will Gossin, Will Colegrove, Ronald Gibbs and the many others at the University of Chicago, the Clinton Foundation, and beyond. You all have helped me become a better social entrepreneur.

Thank you to my roommates who have been beside me through every stage of my recovery, Matthew Gallaghuer, Joe Kensok, Jack Marshall, and Brain Craighead. Thank you to the American Pakistan Foundation, especially Shamila Choudhury and Sahar Khan, for creating a community that looks out for one another. Thank you to my Brazilian Jiu-Jitsu coaches and training partners, Luis Pantoja and Charles Yang, for teaching me the discipline I needed to fight this illness. Thank you to Briana Lopez, Danielle Deiotte, Rahim Rasool, Junaid Ahmed, Margarita Louka, Srishti Gupta, Catherine Dudun, Spencer Asay, Ali Al-Haj, Ali Hussain, and Osama Shahid for simply being present for me whenever I needed you. Thank you to all my well-wishers all over the world who prayed for me and continue to inquire about my recovery.

And finally, Allah kah shukar, thank you God, for giving me another shot at life. I promise to use it well.

Made in the USA
Las Vegas, NV
13 May 2023

72017592R00066